GUIDE TO PREVENTION OF LIFESTYLE DISEASES

LIVE A HEALTHY LIFESTYLE TO FIGHT DISEASES

GUIDE TO PREVENTION OF LIFESTYLE DISEASES

LIVE A HEALTHY LIFESTYLE TO FIGHT DISEASES

Edited by

DR. R. KUMAR
MBBS, MS

and

DR. MEENAL KUMAR
MBBS, MD, DGO

Foreword by

DR. S.K. SHARMA
Director,
PGI, Chandigarh

DEEP & DEEP PUBLICATIONS PVT. LTD.
F-159, Rajouri Garden, New Delhi-110027

GUIDE TO PREVENTION OF LIFESTYLE DISEASES

ISBN 81-7629-518-3

Typeset by S.S. COMPOSERS,
3190, Mohindra Park, Shakur Basti, Delhi-110034.

Printed in India at ELEGANT PRINTERS,
A-38/2, Maya Puri, Phase-I, New Delhi-110064.

Published by DEEP & DEEP PUBLICATIONS PVT. LTD.
F-159, Rajouri Garden, New Delhi-110027.
Phones: 25435369, 25440916
E-mail: ddpbooks@yahoo.co.in • deep98@del3.vsnl.net.in
Showroom:
2/13, Ansari Road, Daryaganj, New Delhi-110002 • Telefax: 23245122

CONTENTS

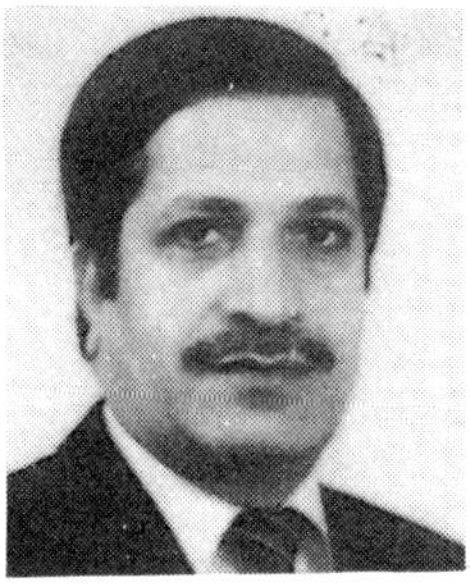

FOREWORD

Our food habits have undergone a sea change and so did our working style and environment. We are caught in a web of faulty eating and sedentary lifestyle. This has resulted in an epidemic of lifestyle diseases, viz. diabetes, obesity, heart disease, cancers, stroke and many more. Now the old classical set of doctors, physicians or surgeons, would not be able to cope with the increasing load of ailments which are life-threatening, disabling and unaffordable in terms of financial outlay required by the society or individual. A new set of doctors have to emerge to look after these lifestyle diseases and thus leading to healthy community, prolong longevity and save the nation's valuable resources and productivity. This also entails increasing the level of public health education and awareness about health and disease. This book, edited by two Chandigarh-based senior clinicians, with contributions from the very best from this region, mostly from PGI, will serve that very purpose.

Dr. R. Kumar, a renowned eye-specialist and health columnist, formerly from PGI, and his wife Dr. Meenal, a senior gyanecologist working under Chandigarh Administration, have taken a leap forward in producing a series of books in public interest on better lifestyle and prevention of disease. Written in simple language and impressive style, this book will serve the purpose of public health education and refreshing the knowledge of family physicians, alike. Such books need encouragement, as valuable tools of health development and prevention of disease, by the Government and NGOs alike.

I am sure Drs. Kumars will continue to serve the community with their endeavors, for a long time to come. I wish them all the success.

S.K. SHARMA,
Director, PGI, Chandigarh

PREFACE

In the coming decades, lifestyle diseases will turn major killers in India. The country is going the way of developed countries like U.S., and researchers fear that by 2012 seven disease groups would drive the growth in the number of out-patients. Cancer, heart ailments, circulatory and nervous disorders, musculo-skeletal diseases, ailments of the sense organs and asthma will make life difficult for an increasing number of people. With increasing stress, stress-related or lifestyle diseases would be on the rise. This clearly establishes the link between changing socio-economic situation and disease pattern. The young hi-flying class in their 30s and 40s will see their lifestyle leading to unimaginable deterioration in their health. This book deals with issues concerning faulty lifestyle and occurrence of major and minor ailments, public awareness, ways of prevention, etc. What is heartening is that most of the lifestyle ailments are preventable.

What exactly are lifestyle ailments? The affluent class follows a style of living that demands activities that may prove to be fatal. Many of the lifestyle ailments owe their origin to work atmosphere, changes in daily routine, eating patterns, sexual permissiveness and the like. For instance, in our highly technical job environment ailments like Carpal Tunnel Syndrome are common. Working on a keyboard for long hours could give your fingers and wrists this ailment. Also, sitting in a very strained position for hours together could prove bad for your spine. There are more in the form of musculo-skeletal uneasiness, ailments of the sense organs and asthma due to the bad air around us. Hectic schedules at work could gift you the dreaded heart ailments and blood pressure. How they affect your health in the long-run needs no elaboration. But then, you are in no position to quit work. You are even unwilling to shed your affluent lifestyle.

Three levels of prevention are now known: *Primary* (Intended to prevent disease among healthy people), *Secondary* (Directed towards those in whom the disease has already developed), *Tertiary* (To reduce the disability consequent to disease). In addition, discoveries in the field of nutrition have added a new dimension to preventive medicine. New strategies have been developed for combating specific deficiencies as for example, nutritional blindness and iodine deficiency disorders. Another notable development in the 20th century and now in the 21st century is the development of "screening" for the diagnosis of disease in its pre-symptomatic stage, e.g. the cholesterol estimation and mammography (to detect proneness to cardiovascular diseases and breast cancer respectively). This approach of pre-emptying the disease or its cause by timely intervention in the lifestyle is of great importance. Similar is the case with cancer cervix and other cancers, where prevention and early detection are the keys to longer and better quality of life.

The risk factors we can treat or modify include:

- Cigarette and tobacco smoke
- High blood cholesterol
- High blood pressure
- Physical inactivity
- Obesity and overweight
- Diabetes mellitus
- Unprotected Sexual contacts

This emphasis on prevention has the potential to produce better health as well as to offer tremendous cost savings.

We are designed to be predominantly vegetarian creatures. Our present culture creates a bounty of meat, dairy products, sweets and fats. As a direct consequence of the above we get increasing skin fold thicknesses, hypertension, coronary artery disease, cancers and many other disabling and killing ailments. For fitness moderate intensity exercises are necessary. What kind of activity is considered to be of moderate intensity? Swimming, brisk walking, riding a bicycle, washing and waxing the car, climbing stairs, and cleaning up the yard.

Avoidance of carcinogenic agents exposure, concerned with lifestyle and consequently, the reduction of cancer risk is possible. As is known, 70% of cancer incidence and mortality could be avoided by healthy lifestyle. At the same time, our population is least informed concerning the carcinogenic agent's exposure and possibilities to reduce the cancer risk.

Women constitute nearly half the country's population. Increased incidence of obesity, diabetes, high blood cholesterol and high blood pressure are largely responsible for ill-health of the women, caused by three major factors: (1) faulty diet of women, consuming too many sweets, fatty and deep-fried food that have a lot of hidden fat, (2) insufficient physical activity, common in majority of middle class and effluent urban women, (3) low nutrition; low calories and low quality of food. It is further pointed out that a large number of women have breast cancer, cancer of the uterine cervix (part of the female genital tract which lies above the vagina) besides high incidence of cancer of the lungs and ovaries, and gall bladder stones. Many women have arthritis. Another disturbing trend about women health is that now more than one-third of heart attack and angina patients are women, between the ages of thirty and forty-five. Till a few decades ago, women never had this disease before the onset of menopause. This is due to more women acquiring smoking habits, becoming job-oriented and having to put up with growing stress of life. Other factors include intake of contraceptive pills. Heart patients and persons suspecting symptoms of heart disease should approach their gynaecologists at the earliest. Counselling includes preventive, therapeutic and curative aspects of the ailments. Regular exercises, better physical and mental environment, besides correct food are other essentials.

This book covers several aspects of lifestyle diseases and their prevention

Chandigarh

DR. R. KUMAR
DR. MEENAL KUMAR

1

PREVENTING DISEASES THROUGH HEALTHY LIFESTYLE

I. INTRODUCTION

The diseases of modern times are not so much due to malnutrition and dangerous infections, but are due to faulty and reckless lifestyle. Though the dream of life long health for all may remain a dream, the lifestyle can be controlled and modified for preventing diseases and improving health. An average Indian eats either low nutrition or high fat diet, depending upon his status as *haves or have-nots*. The *haves* also indulge in high sugar and high salt foods as a symbol of luxury or richness. The urban neo-rich are depending more and more on over-processed foods or fast foods in preference to natural foods such as fruits, vegetables, whole grains, etc. Instead of healthful soups or Soya milk they prefer nutritionally depleted soft drinks and colas as a symbol of modernity or opulence. While he takes very rich non-vegetarian foods in abundance as a part of living in high society, he does not like to move his limbs for most activities. Vehicles that provide the maximum comforts to us all have in fact proved to be the biggest bane of our civilization. With plenty of mutton and chicken and *paranthas* and little exercise, obesity has come as an epidemic for people of all age groups.

1.1 Negative Self-Image

With negative self-image and bouts of frustration and depression, dependence on smoking, alcohol and drugs of abuse the modern youth is becoming a victim of newly acquired prosperity. Dissatisfied with himself/herself and under the influence of 'bold sex wave' sexual activity is being used to achieve numerical targets and to prove or disapprove matters and not for any satisfaction or enjoyment and certainly not for the avowed objective of procreation. Urinary infections and related problems, pelvic inflammations, infertility, cancer cervix are the obvious outcomes. Oscillating between anxiety and depression he stands to degradation: physically, emotionally and spiritually. The postulation that faulty lifestyle leads to disharmony at the level of consciousness, which in turn leads to disease occurrence may not be baseless.

1.2 Environmental Degradation

Our environment has a lot to do with our health and disease. The pollution of various kinds is increasing day in and day out. The toxic gases (emitted by increasing number of vehicles and factories), chemicals, heavy metals, artificial substances, noise, effect our mind and body both and lead to stress on the immune system in a macro as well as micro-manner. The allergies, the infections, the metabolic ailments, the respiratory problems, the asthmatic conditions, the obesity, the constipation and the cancers are only a few of the self-inflicted set of diseases. The other set of ailments is caused by hurry and worry leading to a sense of competition, one-upmanship, overstrain, speed, ambition, anxiety, impatience, lust for money, passions (for sex or substances of euphoria for momentary gratification), addictions, comforts, luxuries, etc.

Presence of a contaminated source, contaminated environmental media (soil, sediment, water, air, biota), a point of exposure (media), an exposure route (ingestion, inhalation, dermal contact), and the presence of a receptor population receiving a dose at a level where health effects may be realized. A person who is exposed to a contaminant may not necessarily develop a disease or ill-health effects. The type of contaminant, the amount received into the body (dose), and how the body reacts will influence disease development. In addition, several other factors may determine whether disease occurs or not and include the age, race, sex, genetics, diet, and other lifestyle factors of an individual. For some diseases, a period of time (20-30 years) may occur between when the individual was exposed to a contaminant and develops the disease. This period of time is termed the "latency period." The development of many cancers involves this latency period. In addition, it is rare that a causal relationship can be determined between exposure to a contaminant and adverse health effects. Usually many factors are involved in the development of a disease, and often not all these factors are known for a population.

1.3 Hurry, Worry, Competition, Oneupmanship

'Never get so busy making a living that you forget to make a life'. This age old saying couldn't have been more timely. A study undertaken by the Confederation of Indian Industry (CII) in association with McKinsey in November 2002 brought to light an alarming situation waiting to hit those caught in the vortex of a competitive world. The study predicted that in the coming decades, lifestyle diseases will turn major killers in India. The country is going the way of developed countries, and researchers fear that by 2012 seven disease groups would drive the growth in the number of out-patients. Cancer, heart ailments, circulatory and nervous disorders, musculo-skeletal diseases, ailments of the sense organs and asthma will take over making life difficult for an increasing number of people. With increasing stress, stress-related or lifestyle diseases would be on the rise. This clearly establishes the link between changing socio-economics and disease pattern. The young hi-flying class in their 30s and 40s will see their lifestyle leading to unimaginable deterioration in their health.

What exactly are lifestyle ailments? The affluent class follows a style of living that demands activities that may prove to be fatal. Many of the lifestyle ailments owe their origin to work atmosphere, changes in daily routine and the like. For instance, in our highly technical job environment ailments like Carpal Tunnel Syndrome are common. Working on a keyboard for long hours could give your fingers and wrists this ailment. Also, sitting in a very strained position for hours together could prove bad for your spine. There are more in the form of musculo-skeletal uneasiness, ailments of the sense organs and asthma due to the bad air around us. Hectic schedules at work could gift you the dreaded heart ailments and blood pressure. How they affect your health in the long run needs no elaboration. But then, you are in no position to quit work. You are even unwilling to shed your affluent lifestyle. In the end, the body is the loser.

Yoga as a form of therapy is worth looking into as a means to check these diseases. However, it is unfortunate that Indians are still hesitant to try simple measures of prevention and are hankering after advanced technologies and techniques. On the other hand, Westerners are now taking to Yoga and Ayurveda in a very big way.

2. PREVENTIVE MEASURES

It has been said that an ounce of prevention is better than a pound of cure. Preventive medicine is applied to "healthy" people; its primary objective is prevention of disease and promotion of health.

समदोषः समाग्निश्च समधातु मलक्रियः ।
प्रसन्न आत्मा इंद्रिय मनः स्वस्थ इति अभिधीयते ।।

"Samadosha samagnisch samadhatu malakriya
Prasanna atma indiria mana swastha iti abhidhiyate."

Having a balanced state of Doshas, Agni (Digestive Fire), Dhatus (tissues) and normal functioning of Mala (waste products), cheerful state of Atma (soul), sensory organs, mind is the symptoms of healthy life.

The eradication of small pox is one of the greatest triumphs of preventive medicine. Anti-rabies treatment, cholera vaccine, diphtheria antitoxin and anti-typhoid vaccine are other notable achievements. There are still many diseases, which are widely prevalent in the tropics such as malaria and leprosy for which vaccines are under development. From the foregoing the impression one gets is that preventive medicine is all about vaccination. Actually preventive medicine goes well beyond that. For example, the strategies in the control of vector borne diseases (e.g., malaria, filariasis, plague) have involved the use of insecticides, which has helped in the control of diseases.

2.1 Health Education

Often most neglected issue is health education. Preventive medicine is currently faced with the problem of "population explosion" in developing countries where population over-growth is causing social, economic, political and environmental problems. Control of this "population explosion" is extremely important. People need to be educated about basic issues like education and sanitation. Provisions for proper sewage disposal, clean drinking water are necessities that should be addressed by the local governing bodies.

2.2 Primary, Secondary and Tertiary Prevention

Three levels of prevention are now known: **Primary** (Intended to prevent disease among healthy people), **Secondary** (Directed towards those in whom the disease has already developed), **Tertiary** (To reduce the disability consequent to disease). In addition, discoveries in the field of nutrition have added a new dimension to preventive medicine. New strategies have been developed for combating specific deficiencies as for example, nutritional blindness and iodine deficiency disorders. Another notable development in the 20th century is the development of "screening" for the diagnosis of disease in its pre-symptomatic stage. For example, the cholesterol estimation and mammography (to detect proneness to cardiovascular diseases and breast cancer respectively), etc. This approach of pre-emptying the disease or its cause by timely intervention in the lifestyle is of great importance. Similar is the case with cancer cervix and other cancers, where prevention and early detection are the keys to longer and better quality of life.

2.3 The Risk Factors

The risk factors we can treat or modify include:

- ❑ Cigarette and tobacco smoke
- ❑ High blood cholesterol
- ❑ High blood pressure
- ❑ Physical inactivity
- ❑ Obesity and overweight
- ❑ Diabetes mellitus

This emphasis on prevention has the potential to produce better health as well as to offer tremendous cost savings. We are designed to be predominantly vegetarian creatures. Our present culture creates a bounty of meat, dairy products, sweets and fats. As a direct consequence of the above we get increasing skin fold thicknesses, hypertension, coronary artery disease, cancers and many other disabling and killing ailments.

A few Basic Errors are given below:

(i) The consumption of smoke and pollutants: The human body needs to breathe clean air and not smoke, chemicals or polluted or stale air.

(ii) The consumption of alcohol, colas and caffeine: The human body needs clean and sterile water.

(iii) The dietary consumption of an abundance of fats, animal proteins and sweets: The human body needs high fibre, whole grains, vegetables and beans and fruits with small amounts of fish, nuts and seeds.

(iv) The neglect of exercise: The human body is designed to be lean and muscular, with active life and avoiding sedentary life and too much comfort. Diseases such as diverticulitis, kidney failure, dialysis, gallstones, diabetes, osteoporosis, hypertension, coronary artery disease, stroke, and numerous cancers, including breast, uterine, prostate and colon cancer, are and can be publicly viewed as virtually preventable with exercise and other measures.

3. SMOKING, DRUGS, ALCOHOL, LIBERAL SEX AND ENVIRONMENTAL ABUSE?

The so-called modern lifestyle has displaced us from the value-based living for the betterment of one's society, family and self to momentary pleasures, irrespective of the consequences thereof. These are not difficult to analyse.

3.1 Smoking

Cigarette smoke contains over 4,000 health-threatening compounds, of which 200 are known poisons. Regardless of the number of toxins, however, there is little doubt about the devastating effect smoking has on one's health. No other consumer product comes close to tobacco in the number of deaths they cause. In the United States, for example, ten times more people die from tobacco-related illnesses than from automobile accidents. The World Health Organization (WHO) estimates that on a global scale, smoking claims three million lives annually. In addition to an increased risk of cancer and heart disease, smokers suffer more frequently from colds, gastric ulcers, chronic bronchitis, and higher blood pressure than non-smokers. Smoking also diminishes one's sense of smell and taste. Clearly, giving up smoking is one of the most important step in preventive health.

3.2 Drugs

Drug abuse has taken an enormous toll on human life worldwide. The U.S. Department of Health and Human Services says: "Every year, drug abuse kills 14,000 Americans." But illicit drug users are not the only ones affected by the drug trade. In order to finance their habit, many addicts turn to violence and a life of crime. Drug abuse, of course, is far from being a problem only in the United States. According to one estimate, every year anywhere from 160,000 to 210,000 people worldwide die from injecting drugs. In addition, millions use other types of harmful drugs.

3.3 Alcohol

While hard drugs like crack cocaine and heroin capture public attention, the abuse of alcohol inflicts much more damage in volume terms. It is toxic to liver and other vital organs, no doubt, it is also an underlying cause of violent crimes and serious vehicular accidents. It keeps the victim and his family famished and malnourished.

3.4 Environmental Abuse

From the public health perspective it is necessary to assess the health loss to environmental exposures, as there are indications that the perception of environmental health risks may be somewhat distorted in our society. To do so one has to apply a public health currency unit that encompasses the very diverse responses that may be associated with environmental pollution. That may range from slight aggravation of respiratory disease all the way up to the loss of many potentially healthy life years due to premature mortality. Our assessment has to comprise important aspects of health such as quantity of life, quality of life and number of people involved. Inspired by the Global burden of disease project we applied a concept very close to the disability adjusted life years (DALYs). At birth we all have eighty years of potentially healthy life ahead. Unfortunately, most of us will suffer from diseases, due to our genetic program, our unhealthy lifestyles, dietary, occupational, environmental factors or just bad luck. How to estimate the loss of DALYs that can be attributed to environmental exposures? Should we concentrate on carcinogenic air pollution or would the abatement of noise exposure provide better returns.

3.5 Liberal Sex

Sex wave has swept away all the boundries of inhibitions. The modern permissive society has made sex too liberal and co-habitation with multiple partners has become more of a norm. The sexually transmitted diseases and some other ailments related to intimate physical touch have spread like wild fire. AIDS, Chlamydia, hepatitis, urinary infections, pelvic inflammations and their complications are only some of the consequences. Safe sex and within the sacrosanct barriers is strongly indicated.

4. IMMUNIZATIONS

This is the single most important area where the timely preventive action can prevent a fatal or disabling disease in the community or individual. This has been the most successful and cost-effective intervention. Let us study some of the vaccines, which have brought a qualitative and quantitative change in the health arena.

4.1 Hepatitis B Vaccine (Hep B)

All infants should receive the first dose of hepatitis B vaccine soon after birth and before hospital discharge; the first dose may also be given by age 2 months if the infant's mother is HBsAg-negative. Only monovalent hepatitis B vaccine can be used for the birth dose. Monovalent or combination vaccine containing Hep B may be used to complete the series; four doses of vaccine may be administered if combination vaccine is used. The second dose should be given at least 4 weeks after the first dose, except for Hib-containing vaccine, which cannot be administered before age 6 weeks. The third dose should be given at least 16 weeks after the first dose and at least 8 weeks after the second dose. The last dose in the vaccination series (third or fourth dose) should not be administered before age 6 months. Infants born to Bag-positive mothers should receive hepatitis B vaccine and 0.5 mL hepatitis B immune globulin (HBIG) within 12 hours of birth at separate sites. The second dose is recommended at age 1-2 months and the vaccination series should be completed (third or fourth dose) at age 6 months. Infants born to mothers whose HBsAg status is unknown should receive the first dose of the hepatitis B vaccine series within 12 hours of birth. Maternal blood should be drawn at the time of delivery to determine the mother's HBsAg status; if the HBsAg test is positive, the infant should receive HBIG as soon as possible (no later than age 1 week).

4.2 Diphtheria and Tetanus Toxoids and Pertussis Vaccine (DTP)

The first 3 doses of DTP vaccine should be administered as per schedule in the first few months of birth. The fourth dose of DTP may be administered as early as age 12 months, provided 6 months have elapsed since the third dose and the child is unlikely to return at age 15-18 months. Tetanus and diphtheria toxoids (Td) is recommended at age 11-12 years if at least 5 years have elapsed since the last dose of tetanus and diphtheria toxoid-containing vaccine. Subsequent routine Td boosters are recommended every 10 years.

4.3 Haemophilus Influenzae Type b (Hib) Conjugate Vaccine

Three Hib conjugate vaccines are licensed for infant use. If PRP-OMP (PedvaxHIB® or ComVax® [Merck]) is administered at ages 2 and 4 months, a dose at age 6 months is not required. DTaP/Hib combination products should not be used for primary immunization in infants at ages 2, 4 or 6 months, but can be used as boosters following any Hib vaccine.

4.4 Inactivated Polio Vaccine (IPV)

An all-IPV schedule is recommended for routine childhood polio vaccination. All children should receive four doses of IPV at ages 2 months, 4 months, 6-18 months, and 4-6 years.

4.5 Measles, Mumps, and Rubella Vaccine (MMR)

The first dose of MMR is given at 12-15 months of age. The second dose of MMR is recommended routinely at age 4-6 years but may be administered during any visit, provided at least 4 weeks have elapsed since the first dose and that both doses are administered beginning at or after age 12 months. Those who have not previously received the second dose should complete the schedule by the 11-12 year old visit.

4.6 Varicella Vaccine

Varicella vaccine is recommended at any visit at or after age 12 months for susceptible children, i.e. those who lack a reliable history of chickenpox. Susceptible persons aged > 13 years should receive two doses, given at least 4 weeks apart.

4.7 Pneumococcal Vaccine

The heptavalent pneumococcal conjugate vaccine (PCV) is recommended for all children age 2-23 months. It is also recommended for certain children age 24-59 months. Pneumococcal polysaccharide vaccine (PPV) is recommended in addition to PCV for certain high-risk groups.

4.8 Hepatitis A Vaccine

Hepatitis A vaccine is recommended for use in selected cases and for certain high-risk groups; consult your local public health authority.

4.9 Influenza Vaccine

Influenza vaccine is recommended annually for children age >= 6 months with certain risk factors (including but not limited to asthma, cardiac disease, sickle cell disease, HIV, diabetes; and can be administered to all others wishing to obtain immunity. Children aged <= 12 years should receive vaccine in a dosage appropriate for their age (0.25 mL if age 6-35 months or 0.5 mL if aged >= 3 years). Children aged <= 8 years who are receiving influenza vaccine for the first time should receive two doses separated by at least 4 weeks.

5. PREVENTIVE GUIDELINES FOR ADULTS

The preventive care will include clinical examination and certain tests to make assessment of various parameters, as per specific needs and situations, e.g. HEMOGLOBIN test should be performed yearly in women with excessive menstrual flow. BLOOD PRESSURE DETERMINATION should be obtained on each clinic visit. Screening should be done every 2 years if normotensive and every year if diastolic BP is 90 over above, patient is obese, black, has a 1st degree family member with hypertension or a personal history of hypertension.

5.1 Mammograms and other Screenings

Screening of breat through mammogram should be done every other year in women 40 to 50 years of age and yearly from 50 to 70 years of age. Similarly, screening for colon cancer for persons with normal risk should begin at age 50 and consist of a flexible sigmoidoscopy every 5 years with fecal occult blood examination annually or a colonoscopy every 10 years. A digital rectal examination should be done with each of these exams.

Screening for diabetes entails plasma glucose estimation every 3 years beginning at age 45. Testing should begin at age 40 and be done every other year if any of the following risk factors are present: family history of diabetes in parents or siblings; obesity (body weight greater than 120% of ideal), high-risk ethnicity (Indian); history of glucose intolerance; hypertension, hyperlipidemia (values for HDL cholesterol <35 mg/dl and/or triglycerides >250 mg/dl), history of gestational diabetes, or one or more infants weighting more than 9 lbs at birth. In known diabetics, the following should be done at least yearly: GLYCOSLATED HEMOGLOBIN, MICROALBUMIN, RETINAL EYE EXAM, FOOT EXAM, LIPID PROFILE, esp. LDL.

Adults (20 years of age and older) should have a fasting lipoprotein profile consisting of a total cholesterol, LDL cholesterol, high-density lipoprotein (HDL) cholesterol, and triglyceride once every 5 years. SCREENING FOR MELANOMA AND SKIN CANCERS should be done every 3 years from age 20 to 39 and yearly after age 40. The patient should be educated regarding sun avoidance and sunscreen use. BONE DENSITY EXAMINATION is recommended on all post-menopausal women who present with fractures or who have one or more additional risk factors for osteoporosis (besides menopause).

5.2 Cervical Cancer Secreening by Regular Pap Tests

Pap test should be performed in all women who are or have been sexually active, and should be instituted after a woman first engages in sexual intercourse. If the sexual history is unknown or considered unreliable, screening should begin at age 18. At least three initial screening tests should be performed one year apart. For women who have had at least three normal annual smears, the screening interval may be lengthened to 3 years except that women at increased risk for cervical cancer should be screened every 2 years. Screening may be discontinued at age 65 if the following criteria are met: the women have been regularly screened, have had two satisfactory smears, and have had no abnormal smears within the previous nine years. For all women over age 65 who have not been previously screened, three normal annual smears should be documented prior to discontinuation of screening. Use of Pap smears is not recommended in women who have had hysterectomies for reasons other than cancer. Annual PSA testing in combination with annual digital rectal examination should be offered to all men aged 50 years and older with a life expectancy of ten years or more. Annual screening should be offered at age 40 to men at high risk for prostate cancer. However, rather than screening all men for prostate cancer as a matter of routine, physicians should describe the potential benefits and known harms of screening, diagnosis, and treatment; listen to the patient's concerns; and then individualize the decision to screen. Testing with tuberculin should be performed every 3-5 years in persons with risk factors for acquiring tuberculosis. These factors are persons infected with HIV, close contacts of persons known or suspected of having tuberculosis, persons with medical conditions that increase the risk of infection, persons with a chest X-ray suggestive of old healed tuberculosis, immigrants from countries with a high prevalence of tuberculosis, medically underserved low-income populations, alcoholics and IV drug users, residents of long-term institutions and persons who work in health care facilities.

5.3 Visual Testing

Beginning at age 40, a comprehensive eye examination by an eye care professional should be performed, including screening for visual acuity and glaucoma. This should be repeated every 2 years. This becomes all the more important when the person is suffering from one or the other systemic disease, viz. diabetes, hypertension, kidney disease, headaches, etc.

5.4 Tetanus and Diphtheria Boosters

Boosters are indicated every 10 years. As an alternate strategy, a single booster at 50 years of age can be given to persons who completed the full primary series. RUBELLA IMMUNIZATION is indicated in All women of child-bearing age who lack documented evidence of immunity or prior immunization. HEPATITIS B IMMUNIZATION should be offered to patients of groups at high risk which include: heterosexual individuals who have had more than one sex partner in the previous 6 months and/or those with a recent episode of a sexually transmitted disease, sexually active homosexual or bisexual male, household contact and sex partners of hepatitis B surface antigen positive persons, injection drug users, health care workers and others at occupational risk hemodialysis patients, hemophiliacs and other recipients of certain blood products.

5.5 Thyroid Function Tests

Measurements of thyroid function by TSH is indicated at age 35 and every 5 years thereafter. It may have to be done often if any symptoms are present.

6. HEART AND BLOOD VESSELS

The idea that the progression of heart disease could be halted and that it can be eventually reversed is a radical idea. The idea has been scientifically proven by years of study. The patients who have undergone the reversal program became better and better without medication or surgery. The Reversal Program is completely based on changes in lifestyle and diet. Seemingly, very simple *do's and don'ts* are therefore sometimes ignored. Complex problems have arisen due to complicated lifestyle. Coronary arteries become clogged with plaque over decades, so it takes time to reverse the block, but the cardiac flow improves remarkably. Severe angina and the incidence of cardiac events can decrease. This is probably because heart disease is not just how much blockage is there in the Coronary artery but how much blood flow your heart is receiving. The "Reversal Program" is not only more compassionate as it would prevent surgery, but it can also lead to substantial cost saving. The cost saved is tremendous if one considers surgery, drugs and sometimes resurgery when the graphs can get blocked again. The program is about living longer and living better. Who wants to live longer if you are not happy? It is because about half of all deaths from heart disease are sudden and unexpected, there's little opportunity for treatment. For people at risk of sudden death, prevention is the only hope.

Dr. Trehan, the famous heart surgeon of India stated, as per the paper reports, that he needs one lakh crores of rupees to provide the infrastructure for surgical treatment of heart ailments. However, by the time the nation could cough up this amount the need to provide infrastructure would increase several folds. So the need is to adopt a healthy lifestyle and prevent heart diseases and not to make arrangements for their surgery and not to improve the faulty lifestyle. If all heart attack-prone people were treated surgically, the cost would be unaffordable for the nation as well as the families concerned. This is even more true for heart transplants. Technological treatments for heart disease such as angioplasty, thrombolytic therapy, antiarrhythmic drugs and pacemakers aren't cures. More importantly, such procedures can do nothing about slowing arteriosclerosis for future, the underlying process that causes heart disease. Arteriosclerosis begins in young adulthood, but it may be decades before clinical disease shows up. So the symptoms would come back after a variable period, despite the palliative interventions.

6.1 Exercise

Exercise does help in prevention of heart disease as it conditions your heart, but only if done on a regular basis. The exercise that you can do most simply is called "The 5—5s." This walking program starts by walking 2½ minutes out and 2½ minutes back from your home, once per day. This is 5 minutes per day, which you do 5 days per week. Every Monday, add 5 minutes (add 2½ minutes out, and add 2½ minutes back), so that you are walking for 10 minutes daily the second week, 15 minutes daily the third week, and so on. Your goal is to work up to 50 minutes per day, 5 days a week, 50 weeks a year. (Holidays and vacations are your two weeks off.) This is an ideal outdoors exercise that can be done in all seasons if you just have the determination and dress correctly. For more fit and younger people moderate intensity exercises can also be done. What kind of activity is considered to be of moderate intensity? Swimming, brisk walking, riding a bicycle, washing and waxing the car, climbing stairs and cleaning up the yard. You don't need to join a gym or a health club to safeguard your health. Medical authorities recommend that if you have a history of cardiovascular disease or if you are a male over 40 years of age or a female over 50, you should be sure to consult your doctor before starting any exercise program

Our biology would thrive on a high fiber, whole-food, nearly vegetarian, 10% to 20% diet, with foods such as brown rice, whole grain pasta, stone-ground breads, boiled or steamed vegetables, fruits, bean dishes, nuts and seeds, and far less meat and poultry, white-flour breads and pasta and dairy products.

Dr. Steven Blair, an editor of the U.S. surgeon general's report on physical fitness, says: "People who go from a sedentary lifestyle to moderate activity cut their heart disease mortality rate in half." Sadly, many people today do not engage in even moderate physical activity. Previously it was thought that only vigorous aerobic exercise brought health benefits. But strenuous workouts are not necessary to improve fitness. In fact, "burning as few as 150 calories a day [by mild exercise] can reduce the risk of heart disease, high blood pressure, cancer and diabetes". When you select an exercise activity, it is important to choose something that you enjoy doing. Otherwise, you will not make it a part of your life-style. The key is not so much *what* you do for exercise but *how often* you do it. The U.S. National Institutes of Health suggests that as a general guideline, "children and adults alike should set a goal of accumulating at least 30 minutes of moderate-intensity physical activity on most, and preferably all, days of the week."

6.2 High Calorie Diet

It seems unlikely that the human body will be benefited from a high calorie diet that contains 30% fat or, much sugar or artificial Sweeteners or too much salt. So, if your habit is to consume a diet high in calories, fatty foods (meat and poultry, dairy products, fast and fried foods), and white-flour baked goods and low in whole, fiber rich foods (fruits, vegetables, beans and whole grains), then you are a candidate for trouble. These dietary habits cause Coronary artery disease. Any of these "unhealthy" foods can be eaten once in a while, but to consume them regularly increases the risk of developing cancer, heart disease, diabetes and other diseases.

6.3 Atrial Fibrillation

If you have atrial fibrillation, the upper left chamber of your heart beats rapidly and unpredictably, making it hard for all the blood in the chamber to empty. The remaining blood tends to form clots that can travel to any part of your body. If they travel to the brain, these clots can cause a stroke. Treatment with anticoagulants (or blood-thinners) such as aspirin can prevent these clots from forming. The most recent clinical studies have shown that warfarin is superior to aspirin in preventing stroke. However, Warfarin may increase the risk of bleeding. Careful regular monitoring of blood levels and proper dosage should keep this risk in check. Most bleeding incidents are preventable and treatable.

6.4 Carotid Artery Disease

The carotid arteries run through the neck and supply blood to the brain. When the walls of the carotid arteries are narrowed by fatty deposits known as plaque, small clots in the blood can cut-off blood supply to the brain and cause a stroke. A surgical procedure known as a carotid endarterectomy clears arteries of plaque. If you have had a minor stroke or symptoms that suggest you are at high risk for a stroke, and there is evidence of severe blockage in your carotid arteries, your health care provider may suggest you consider carotid endarterectomy as a preventive procedure.

Certain tests may be required to confirm the diagnosis of carotid artery disease, e.g. angiography, Magnetic resonance imaging (MRI) and ultrasonic color Doppler studies. Carotid endarterectomy carries some risks. There can be complications if parts of the plaque break away during the procedure and block an artery to the brain or if artery incisions leak.

6.5 Taking Aspirin

If you are at risk for a heart attack, taking aspirin every day or every other day can lower your risk. You may be at higher risk for a heart attack if you can say yes to any of the following: a man over 40, a woman past menopause. Smoker, diabetic, high blood pressure, high cholesterol, or a family history of heart disease. Taking aspirin is safe. But for some people, aspirin can increase the chance of bleeding in the stomach or intestines.

7. STROKE PREVENTION

Stroke occurs when blood flow to the brain is blocked, either by narrowed blood vessels or blood clots or when there is bleeding in the brain. Deprived of nutrients, brain nerve cells begin to die within a few minutes. As a result, stroke can cause vision and sensory loss, problems with walking and talking, or difficulty in thinking clearly. In many cases, the effects of stroke are irreversible. Some people are more at risk for stroke than others. Chronic health conditions such as high blood pressure and diabetes can increase your risk, as well as lifestyle choices such as smoking cigarettes, being overweight, or drinking excessively. Men, African Americans, and people with a family history of stroke have a higher risk as well. If you have already had a stroke or a transient ischemic attack (referred to as a TIA or "mini-stroke"), you are at highest risk. Warning signs include sudden unexplained numbness or tingling (especially on one side), slurred speech, blurred vision, stumbling, or clumsiness.

Experts now believe that stroke is as preventable as heart attack. In addition to primary prevention tactics such as quitting smoking, drinking only in moderation, and exercising, there are medical interventions that can decrease your risk of stroke if you are in a high-risk group. Recent studies show that if you have conditions known as atrial fibrillation or carotid artery disease, there are interventions that can dramatically lower your risk of stroke.

8. CANCER PREVENTION

Risk for each person to get cancer straightly correlates with one's lifestyle, food, occupation, living and resting place and environment pollution by carcinogenic agents. Carcinogenic agents are divided in 3 groups:

- Physical carcinogenic agents (ionizing radiation, sun ultraviolet rays, electric-magnetic fields);
- Chemical carcinogenic agents (anthropogenic chemical substances); and
- Biological carcinogenic agents (viruses and bacteria).

Carcinogenic agents exposure on population is possible due to following ways:

- Air (occupational place, outdoor, building);
- Drinking and irrigating water;
- Atmospheric precipitations (direct exposure of radioactive rains, pollution of soil and consequently agricultural products by radioactive and chemical carcinogenic agents, etc.);
- Meals and non-alcoholic drinks;
- Widely used everyday products (chewing gums, soap, detergents, medications, perfumery, etc.). Carcinogenic agent's exposure on population could be realized by the following ways, concerned with lifestyle;
- Active and passive (environmental) tobacco smoking;
- Alcoholic drinks;
- Drug addiction;
- Non-controlled sexual life; and
- Natural and artificial tan.

8.1 Primary Prevention

Avoidance of carcinogenic agents exposure, concerned with lifestyle and consequently, the reduction of cancer risk is possible due to healthy lifestyle. As is known, 70% of cancer incidence and mortality could be avoided by healthy lifestyle. At the same time, our population is least adequately informed concerning the carcinogenic agent's exposure and possibilities to reduce the cancer risk due to healthy lifestyle and adoption of health habits. (See Appendix at page 270)

The lack of appropriate legislative basis, which can ensure the law-based conduction of population social defense, is also very important issue. It will promote the protection of population from carcinogenic agent's exposure, support to maintain their health status and/or make them healthier, consequently increase the mean life time and faster the country social-economical development.

Numerous cancer etiologic factors are already identified at the present time and cancer primary prevention is possible due to avoiding their exposure on humans. The main point of National Model of Cancer Prevention consists the avoidance of exposure of all already identified cancer etiologic factors due to all available at the present time measures, or at least their reglamentation by adoption of legislation basis with conductive intersectional economic mechanisms.

It's necessary to conduct activities aimed at creating of favourable environment, which means the protection of environment, atmospheric and working place air, soul, water, sea, flora, dietary products, etc.) from pollution by chemical, radioactive and biologic (viruses, bacteria, etc.), carcinogenic agents. Popularization of healthy lifestyle to public at large, through the following means:

1. Banning of Tobacco smoking at state and non-state organizations and places of public meeting;
2. Ban the Advertisement of tobacco products (as one of the type of health hazardous narcotic means) and strong alcoholic drinks;
3. Advertisement banning of non-alcoholic drinks and other dietary products without the testing on carcinogenic agents and appropriate certification; and
4. Regulate the manufacture, export and import of dietary products, non-alcoholic and alcoholic drinks and other consuming products without obligating testing on carcinogenic agents and certification.

8.2 Ways of Occupation Cancer Prevention

- Acceptance of working place air hygienic standards in order to defend the staff members from professional cancer development;

- Manufacturers' owners and managers should be obligated to ensure sanitary-hygienic security and promote the industry (factory, enterprise, etc.) technological improvement, which will be directed to maintain working place hygienic standards. Due to this, it will be possible to reduce or maximally minimize the exposition of health-hazardous toxic substances (carcinogenic among of them), contained in industrial air and dust (carcinogenic loading);
- Implementation of working place air hygienic standards monitorial control;
- Acceptance of fines in case of working place air hygienic standards violation;
- Acceptance of hygienic guides (admitted border doses and concentrations on each carcinogenic agent) followed by establishment of appropriate fines and monitorial control, which aims the defense of industrial place's and surrounding territory's Eco-systems (atmospheric and working place air, soul, water, flora, etc.) from pollution by carcinogenic agents and toxic industrial products; and
- Considering the fact that the problems are concerned with multiple spheres and sections, work out of real conductive intersectional mechanisms, also communication and explanation of decisions to public at large, is very essential. This will require a suitable legislation on the part of the Government and a community campaign on the part of the public.

8.3 Tobacco and other Intoxicants are the Culprits

"The greatest menace in the world isn't a disease," says *World Watch* magazine, "it's a product." The magazine adds: "Within 25 years, tobacco-induced illness is expected to overtake infectious disease as the leading threat to human health worldwide." Moreover, *Scientific American* says: "An astonishing 30 percent of fatal cancers can be blamed primarily on smoking, and an equal number on lifestyle, especially dietary practices and lack of exercise." Medical authorities recommend that we eat a wide variety of foods, with the largest portion of our calories coming from complex carbohydrates, especially those found in whole grains, beans, vegetables, and fruits. However, our health is affected not only by what we eat but also by how much we eat. It is important to eat in moderation, even to prevent cancers. In recent years much attention has been given to the matter of dietary fat. Many health professionals state that a diet high in saturated fats raises the risk of certain types of cancers. This does not mean, however, that we need to eliminate all fat from our diet. Dietitians suggest that you can soften the impact of making adjustments to your diet by phasing out unhealthy foods gradually. For example, balance your diet over the course of a week, not just one day. If you presently eat red meat every day, try cutting back to three times a week. The same goes for foods high in saturated fats, such as butter, cheese, ice cream, and high-fat snack foods. The goal should be to reduce your intake of fat so that it represents no more than 20 percent of your total calories. A healthy lifestyle also includes a program of regular exercise.

8.4 Carcinogens

Viruses linked with human malignancies include human papillomaviruses (cervical carcinoma), cytomegalovirus (Kaposi's sarcoma), Epstein-Barr virus (Burkitt's lymphoma, immunoblastic lymphoma, and nasopharyngeal carcinoma), and hepatitis B virus (hepatocellular carcinoma). Human retroviruses have been linked to T-cell lymphomas (human T-cell lymphotrophic virus, which have a predilection for skin and bone involvement, hypercalcemia, and a leukemic phase. HIV types I and II are pathogenically linked to AIDS. Patients with AIDS are predisposed to Kaposi's sarcoma and lymphoma, which may be viral in origin.

Of parasites, *Schistosoma haematobium* has been linked to bladder cancer, which usually develops after chronic inflammation and fibrosis. *Opisthorchis sinensis* has been linked to carcinoma of the pancreas and bile ducts.

Chemical carcinogenesis is a multistep process: (1) In initiation, a cell that experiences a carcinogenic event can potentially develop into a neoplastic clone. (2) In promotion, which is reversible, continued existence of the neoplastic clonal proliferation depends on a chemical or agent with little carcinogenic activity. (3) In progression, irreversible growth of altered (neoplastic) cells occurs. An agent that possesses little or no carcinogenic potency (a cocarcinogen) enhances the carcinogenic effect of another agent when exposure is simultaneous. Chemical carcinogenesis is influenced by age, endocrine status, diet, other exogenous agents (cocarcinogens or promoters), and immunologic status. Ultraviolet radiation is a definite cause of skin cancer (i.e., basal and squamous cell carcinoma, melanoma, and especially in xeroderma pigmentosum).

Ionizing radiation is carcinogenic, e.g., survivors of the atomic bomb drop in Hiroshima and Nagasaki have a higher-than-expected incidence of leukemia and several other cancers. Similarly, when ionizing radiation in the form of X-rays is used to treat non-malignant disease (acne, thymic or adenoid enlargement, and ankylosing spondylitis), the incidence of cancer increases, including acute and chronic leukemias; Hodgkin's and non-Hodgkin's lymphomas; multiple myeloma; aplastic anemia terminating in acute non-lymphocytic leukemia (ANLL); myelofibrosis; melanoma; and thyroid cancer. Industrial exposure (e.g., to uranium by mine workers) is linked to development of lung cancer after a 15- to 20-yr latency. Long-term exposure to occupational irradiation or to internally deposited thorium dioxide predisposes persons to angiosarcomas and ANLL.

Chronic irritation to skin leads to chronic dermatitis and on rare occasions ultimately to squamous cell carcinoma.

8.5 Some Do's and Don'ts

1. Control your life, work out healthy diet habits,
2. Increase fruits, vegetables and fiber in your diet,
3. Significanthy reduce in your diet the animal fat, smoked, conserved and salted food,
4. Control your weight,
5. Treat your body by exercises, sport and water procedures,

6. Quit tobacco smoking,
7. Deny adultery,
8. Go easy with alcohol,
9. Deny narcotics, and
10. Avoid the exaggerated tanning by sun rays.

9. PSYCHOSOMATIC DISEASES

Negative thoughts of hatred, jealousy and anger act as slow poison. On the other hand, thoughts of love, compassion and charity are the nectars of life. We are seeing a crisis of humanity, never witnessed before. We have no time to assess our own feelings, emotions and our real needs. We strain ourselves to such an extent that we realize too late that we had been abusing ourselves all these years. Hurry and rush are the order of the day. We are being keyed up with nervous tension and prolongations of our hectic days exhaust us completely. Worry, overwork, fatigue affect us either singly or in combination. Moreover, by deliberately indulging in habits that are totally unsavory for health we are in a collision course with nature. We rest at wrong time, stuff ourselves with wrong foods and spoil our health by drinking, smoking and taking drugs.

9.1 Breakdown under Stress

More and more modern medical and behavioural studies are revealing that a physical breakdown under stress does not necessarily occur only because of causes imposed from outside a person such as genes, infections and environmental agents combined with exhaustion or physical trauma. It can also be due to the life experiences, thoughts, emotions, and behaviour and personality structure. Particular personality types breakdown in specific and predictable ways in times of stress. These breakdowns are manifested when one's life is threatened or is in chronically uncomfortable conditions. Among the growing list is cancer, asthma, migraine, ulcers, hay fever, accident-proneness, infectious diseases, chronic low back pain, temporary blindness, urinary tract infections, Parkinson's disease and multiple sclerosis.

9.2 Childhood Experiences

Interesting studies reveal how experiences, thoughts, emotions and behaviour in childhood can alter the body so that it can be easily affected by different illnesses, later in adult life. Helplessness and hopelessness have been shown to impair the body's immune system, whereas a positive approach does not have this effect. Depression and grief are also known to depress the immune system. Powerful negative emotions causing undue stress can switch on many diseases, which can act on the hypothalamus of the brain and then can affect the body's sympathetic system, the pituitary gland and the immune system. Psychological stress has also been found to raise the level of cholesterol leading to heart attack. Anxiety increases the production of stomach acid leading to ulcer. Psychological stress is known to trigger asthma attacks via the vagus nerve. Thus, the concept of psychosomatic medicine has gained ground in this decade much more than at any other time. The word psychosomatic is derived from two Greek words—psyche (soul) and soma (body)—and it indicates the influence of mind on body and physical health.

10. WOMEN'S HEALTH

Women constitute nearly half the country's population. Increased incidence of obesity, diabetes, high blood cholesterol and high blood pressure are largely responsible for ill-health of the women, caused by three major factors: (1) faulty diet of women, consuming too many sweets, fatty and deep-fried food which have a lot of hidden fat, (2) insufficient physical activity, common in majority of middle class and effluent urban women, (3) low nutrition; low calories and low quality of food. Health problems arise largely on account of a faulty lifestyle which needs to be corrected. It is pointed out that a large number of women have breast cancer, cancer of the uterine cervix (part of the female genital tract which lies above the vagina) besides high incidence of cancer of the lungs and ovaries, and gall bladder stone. Many women have arthritis. Another disturbing trend about women health is that now more than one-third of heart attack and angina patients are women, between the ages of thirty and forty-five. Till a few decades ago, women never had this disease before the onset of menopause. This is due to more women acquiring smoking habits, becoming job-oriented and having to put up with growing stress of life. Other factors include intake of contraceptive pills by prone women. Heart patients and persons suspecting symptoms of heart disease should approach their gynaecologists at the earliest. Counseling includes preventive, therapeutic and curative aspects of the ailments. Regular exercises, better physical and mental environment, besides correct food are other essentials.

10.1 Breast Cancer

Breast cancer continues to be the most commonly diagnosed cancer among women in the United States. In the year 2000, an estimated 183,000 U.S. women were newly diagnosed with breast cancer, and nearly 41,000 women died from the disease. Substantial progress has been made in diagnosing and treating breast cancer. The number of women dying from breast cancer increased slightly in the 1980s, but overall breast cancer deaths have now begun to decline. The 5-year relative survival rate for all women with breast cancer is 85 percent; the 5-year survival rate for women with localized breast cancer is now 96.5 percent.

It is known that black women are more likely than white women to be diagnosed with breast cancer at a later stage after it has spread, they often lack access to state-of-the-art care, often they must overcome barriers associated with poverty and cultural differences, and they may encounter provider biases as well. Research continues into whether black women are at greater risk genetically for more aggressive tumors.

10.2 Cervical Cancer

In 1999, there were an estimated 12,800 cases of invasive cervical cancer in U.S. women, and about 4,800 women died from the disease. Cervical cancer occurs most often among minority women, particularly Asian-American. Although deaths from cervical cancer have declined substantially over the past 30 years, the cervical cancer death rate for black women continues to be more than twice that of white women.

The chance of dying of cervical cancer increases as women get older. Worldwide, cervical cancer is the second or third most common cancer among women, and in some developing countries like India, it is the most common cancer.

Many women still do not have regular Pap tests, particularly older women, uninsured women, minorities, poor women, and women living in rural areas. About half of the women with newly diagnosed invasive cervical cancer have not had a Pap test in the previous 5 years.

- Physicians' preferences help determine treatment for older women with breast cancer.
- Disabled women who have trouble walking are less likely than other women to receive Pap tests and mammograms.
- Hormone replacement therapy does not appear to increase risk of breast cancer recurrence.
- Cervical smears of previously screened post-menopausal women are poor predictors of cervical cancer.
- Community programs are an effective way to reach poor and minority women with health messages.
- Attitudes about mammography affect appointment keeping.
- Women with chronic diseases are less likely than other women to be screened.
- Prophylactic mastectomy may provide substantial gains in life expectancy for women with cancer-disposing genes.

11. PREVENTING MEDICAL ERRORS

Medical errors are one of the Nation's leading causes of death and injury. A recent report by the Institute of Medicine estimates that as many as 44,000 to 98,000 people die in U.S. hospitals each year as the result of medical errors. The Indian figures are not available, but must be much higher than U.S., seeing widespread ignorance, illiteracy, apathy and callousness on the part of patients as well medical care providers. This means that many people die from medical errors as they do with motor vehicle accidents, breast cancer, or AIDS. Medical errors happen when something that was planned as a part of medical care doesn't work out, or when the wrong plan was used in the first place. Medical errors can occur anywhere in the health care system:

- Hospitals.
- Clinics.
- Outpatient Surgery Centers.
- Doctors' Offices.
- Nursing Homes.
- Pharmacies.
- Patients' Homes.

They can happen during even the most routine tasks, such as when a hospital patient on a salt-free diet is given a high-salt meal. Most errors result from problems created by today's complex health care system. But errors also happen when doctors and their patients have problems communicating. For example, a recent study supported by the Agency for Healthcare Research and Quality (AHRQ) found that doctors often do not do enough to help their patients make informed decisions. Uninvolved and uninformed patients are less likely to accept the doctor's choice of treatment and less likely to do what they need to do to make the treatment work. The single most important way you can help to prevent errors is to be an active member of your health care team. That means taking part in every decision about your health care. Research shows that patients who are more involved with their care tend to get better results.

11.1 Medicines

Make sure that all of your doctors know about everything you are taking. This includes prescription and over-the-counter medicines, and dietary supplements such as vitamins and herbs. At least once a year, bring all of your medicines and supplements with you to your doctor. This can help you and your doctor talk about them and find out if there are any problems. It can also help your doctor keep your records up-to-date, which can help you get better quality care.

Make sure your doctor knows about any allergies and adverse reactions you have to medicines. This can help you avoid getting a medicine that can harm you. When your doctor writes you a prescription, make sure you can read it. If you can't read your doctor's handwriting, your pharmacist might not be able to read either. Ask for information about your medicines in terms you can understand—both when your medicines are prescribed and when you receive them. What is the medicine for?

- ❑ How am I supposed to take it, and for how long?
- ❑ What side effects are likely? What do I do if they occur?
- ❑ Is this medicine safe to take with other medicines or dietary supplements I am taking?
- ❑ What food, drink, or activities should I avoid while taking this medicine?

If you know what might happen, you will be better prepared if it does—or, if something unexpected happens instead. That way, you can report the problem right away and get help before it gets worse. A study found that written information about medicines could help patients recognize problem side effects and then give that information to their doctor or pharmacist. When you are being discharged from the hospital, ask your doctor to explain the treatment plan you will use at home. This includes learning about your medicines and finding out when you can get back to your regular activities. Research shows that at discharge time, doctors they should or should not do when they return home. If you are having think their patients understand more than they really do about what surgery, make sure that you, your doctor, and your surgeon all agree and are clear on exactly what will be done. Doing surgery at the wrong site (for example, operating on the left knee instead of the right) is rare. But even once is too often. It is a good idea to find out why a test or treatment is needed and how it can help you. You could be better-off without it.

12. DECIDING TO TAKE MEDICINES

Taking medicines is not always as simple as swallowing a pill. It can involve many steps and decisions each day. Whether you are using a medicine yourself or helping a child or an adult, it is easy to get-off track. Perhaps you:

- ❑ Did not take all of your medicine because you started feeling better.
- ❑ Did not have a prescription filled or refilled (and did not tell your doctor).
- ❑ Forgot to take one or more doses a day.
- ❑ Took more or less medicine than your doctor told you to take.

Work with your health care professionals before, during, and after taking medicines—to give and get information, and to get help if you need it.

12.1 Why should you take this Active Role?

1. Because using medicines in the right way is very important to your health. With proper use of medicines, you can:
   - ❑ Get the medicine's full benefits. For example, if you take too little of a medicine to lower your cholesterol level, you will not reduce your cholesterol as much as you could.
   - ❑ Avoid dangerous problems. Some people end up at a hospital emergency room because they took too much or too little of a medicine, took it the wrong way, or mixed the wrong medicines, foods and drinks. Improper medicine use can make you worse instead of better.
   - ❑ Reduce your chances of having side effects.
2. Because decisions you make about your medicines can affect your schedule, your diet, your finances, and other parts of your daily life.
3. Because most medicine problems can be avoided or

solved—if you talk with your health care professional about what is happening.

12.2 How to Get Involved?

Taking an active role in medicine use is a three-step process:

1. Take part in decisions about your treatment.
2. Follow your treatment plan.
3. Watch for problems and get help in solving them.

When Mona's doctor told her she had high blood pressure, she asked what she could do to lower it. While blood pressure control was important to her, so were other things—like not being bothered by medicine side effects when at work. Mona talked about her concerns, and she also told her doctor about the medicines she takes for her arthritis. Together, they came up with a plan, she felt she could follow, which included a new medicine and some changes in her diet.

Take part in your treatment decisions. Do not be afraid to ask questions and talk about your concerns. You may want to write down questions to ask at your next visit. By taking a moment to ask questions now, you may avoid problems later. Here are some points to cover each time a new medicine is prescribed. Ask: About all parts of your treatment, including diet changes, exercise and medicines. About the risks and benefits of each medicine or other treatment you might get. How often you or your doctor will have to check your medicine's effects. For example, this means checking your cholesterol level if you are taking a medicine to lower it. While asking questions, it is one's duty to give all the information to the doctor, i.e.:

(i) All the medicines you are already taking. This includes prescription medicines and the medicines you buy over the counter, like aspirin or laxatives. Then your doctor can avoid giving you a new medicine that may not work well with one you take now.

(ii) What is important to you about your medicines?

You may want a medicine with the fewest side effects, or the fewest doses to take each day. You may care most about cost, or how the medicine might affect how you live or work. Or, you may want the medicine your doctor believes will work the best. Telling your doctor will help him or her select the best treatment for you.

(iii) If cost is a concern. There may be a generic drug or another lower cost medicine you can take.

(iv) If you have any medicine allergies, or if you have had troubling side effects from a medicine.

(v) If you are or might become pregnant, or if you are nursing a baby.

(vi) Any illnesses or problems for which another doctor or health professional is treating you.

Do not be afraid to "bother" your doctor with your concerns and questions. You need to understand and feel comfortable with your treatment plan.

12.3 Follow your Treatment Plan

To follow the treatment plan you and your doctor agree on, ask questions and tell your health professionals your needs and concerns. The doctor may start by giving you some directions for taking the medicine. Use the list located in this document under "Questions to Ask About Your Medicine" to write down answers you receive about the medicine. If you need more information, you can ask your doctor, pharmacist, or nurse. The name of the medicine and what it is supposed to do. How and when to take the medicine, how much to take, and for how long. What food, drinks, other medicines, or activities you should avoid while taking the medicine. What side effects the medicine may have, and what to do if they occur. If you can get a refill, and how often. About any terms or directions you do not understand. What to do if you miss a dose. If there is written information you can take home. But remember: Your medicine was prescribed for *you*. Never share your prescription medicines with anyone.

12.4 Watch for Problems and Get Help in Solving Them

Keep working with your health professionals while you are taking your medicine. Ask: About the results of medical tests that show how the medicine is working. For example, if you are taking a drug for high blood pressure, what is your blood pressure reading now? Any problems you are having taking your medicine. About side effects or any new problems that may be related to the medicine. Any new medicines that another doctor gave you, and any over-the-counter medicines that you started taking since your last doctor's visit. Before you visit your doctor, make a list of all medicines that you take, try to keep this list up-to-date. How you are feeling since you started taking the medicine. Do you think it is helping?

A yearly medicine check-up is a good way to spot hidden problems. Schedule a time with your doctor to look at all the prescription and over-the-counter medicines you take. They can check for duplicate medicines and proper doses. They can also advice you on medicines that are no longer needed, and tell you how to safely get rid of old medicines.

12.5 Stay Involved

Remember, medicines can only help you if you take them the right way. Follow these important steps each time your doctor prescribes a medicine: Take part in decisions about your treatment. Follow your treatment plan. Watch for problems, and get help in solving them.

13. IF YOU DECIDE TO UNDERGO SURGERY

Are you facing surgery? You are not alone. Millions of Americans have surgery each year. Most operations are not emergencies. This means you have time to ask your surgeon questions about the operation and time to decide whether to have it, and if so, when and where. The information presented here does not apply to emergency surgery. The most important questions to ask about elective surgery are why the procedure is necessary for you and what alternatives there are to surgery. If you do not need to have the operation, then you can avoid any risks that might result. All surgeries and alternative treatments have risks and benefits. They are only worth doing if the benefits are greater than the risks.

Your primary care doctor, that is, your regular doctor, may be the one who suggests that you have surgery and may recommend a surgeon. You may want to identify another independent surgeon to get a second opinion.

13.1 The Questions that Arise

Following are the questions to ask your primary care doctor and surgeon before you have surgery, and the reasons for asking them. Patients who are well informed about their treatment tend to be more satisfied with the outcome or results of their treatment.

Ask your surgeon to explain the surgical procedure. For example, if something is going to be repaired or removed, find out why it is necessary to do so. Your surgeon can draw a picture or a diagram and explain to you the steps involved in the procedure. There are many reasons to have surgery. Some operations can relieve or prevent pain. Others can reduce a symptom of a problem or improve some body function. Some surgeries are performed to diagnose a problem. Surgery also can save your life. Your surgeon will tell you the purpose of the procedure. Ask your surgeon what you will gain by having the operation. For example, a hip replacement may mean that you can walk again with ease. Ask how long the benefits are likely to last. For some procedures, it is not unusual for the benefits to last for a short time only. There might be a need for a second operation at a later date. For other procedures, the benefits may last a lifetime.

When finding out about the benefits of the operation, be realistic. Sometimes patients expect too much and are disappointed with the outcome or results. All operations carry some risk. This is why you need to weigh the benefits of the operation against the risks of complications or side effects.

Complications can occur around the time of the operation. Complications are unplanned events, such as infection, too much bleeding, reaction to anesthesia, or accidental injury. Some people have an increased risk of complications because of other medical conditions. In addition, there may be side effects after the operation. For the most part, side effects can be anticipated. For example, your surgeon knows that there will be swelling and some soreness at the site of the operation.

13.2 Second Opinion

Getting a second opinion from another doctor is a very good way to make sure having the operation is the best alternative for you. If you get one, make sure to get your records from the first doctor so that the second one does not have to repeat tests. One way to reduce the risks of surgery is to choose a surgeon who has been thoroughly trained to do the procedure and has plenty of experience doing it. You can ask your surgeon about his or her recent record of successes and complications with this procedure. Find out where your operation will be performed. Have many of the operations you are thinking about having been done in this hospital? Some operations have higher success rates if they are done in hospitals that do many of those procedures. Until recently, most surgery was performed on an in-patient basis and patients stayed in the hospital for one or more days. Today, a lot of surgery is done on an out-patient basis. Out-patient surgery is less expensive because you do not have to pay for staying in a hospital room.

13.4 Anesthesia

Anesthesia is used so that surgery can be performed without pain. Your surgeon can tell you whether the operation calls for local, or general anesthesia, and why this form of anesthesia is recommended for your procedure. *Local anesthesia* numbs only a part of your body for a short period of time, for example, a tooth and the surrounding gum. *General anesthesia* numbs your entire body for the entire time of the surgery. You will be unconscious if you have general anesthesia. Anesthesia is quite safe for most patients and is usually administered by a specialized physician. If you decide to have an operation, ask to meet with the person who will give you anesthesia. Find out what his or her qualifications are. Ask what the side effects and risks of having anesthesia are in your case. Be sure to tell him or her what medical problems you have including allergies and any medications you have been taking, since they may affect your response to the anesthesia. Your surgeon can tell you how you might feel and what you will be able to do or not do the first few days, weeks, or months after surgery. Ask how long you will be in the hospital. Ask when you can start regular exercise again and go back to work. You do not want to do anything that will slow down the recovery process. Lifting a 10-pound bag may not seem to be "too much" a week after your operation, but it could be.

14. CHILDREN AND YOUTHS ALSO NEED BETTER LIFESTYLE

Expand the disease orientation of health services research to include a focus on children and youths health development.

1. Establish child-sensitive standards for setting research priorities.
2. Increase the size and capacity of the workforce.
3. Develop appropriate laboratories to study child health care.
4. Improve coordination of research funding across the Governments, foundations, and the private sector.
5. Enhance the research function of health care delivery in the private sector.

In 2000, children and adolescents under age 18 had over 212 million ambulatory health care visits, including 49 million visits to hospital out-patients and emergency departments. Only 15 percent of visits to physicians' offices were for well-child care, while a high number of visits were for acute care. Fifty-four percent of visits to hospital emergency departments by 5-14 years old are due to injuries, and injuries are the leading cause of death among those 1-24 years old in the US and other countries. Thus, the focus has to be on acute care and injuries and on the effectiveness, quality, and costs of care for children and adolescents. Researchers have begun to target studies at the distinctive health care needs of adolescents. Establishing healthy behaviours early can reduce risks of acquiring many diseases, e.g. screening for sexually transmitted diseases and smoking cessation.

This quality improvement (QI) intervention addresses provider and system-level barriers to delivery of preventive services to adolescents during primary care visits. The goal is to determine whether a system intervention in a managed health care organization—including provider training and customized screening and charting tools—results in increased delivery of clinical preventive services to adolescents than the usual standard of care.

2

LIFESTYLE AND CANCERS

B.D. Gupta

The primary purpose of this Chapter is to discuss the lifestyles and cancer leading to strategy for primary cancer prevention programme and also to describe some of the criteria for healthy practice through education and promote health-maintaining behaviour to prevent illness. Primary prevention in health care is also important in the area of weight control, diet and exercise. We know that consumption of fat and protein in diet and low intake of fibre has been associated with cancer of the breast, colon, prostate and also uterus. It has been observed and reported that dietary fibre is believed to be a protective factor in the reduction of several cancers including colon. It is also believed and in several studies it has been demonstrated that fruits particularly citrus fruits and vegetables containing Vitamins A and C may be protective and reduce the incidence of cancer. We also want to discuss the use of tobacco particularly chewing of tobacco in various forms including the recent introduction of a mixture of

* Professor Emeritus of Radiotherapy and Oncology, Post-graduate Institute of Medical Education and Research, (PGI), Chandigarh.

pan masala with and without tobacco. It is also discussed in several fora and meetings that use of pan masala alone is directly related to the high incidence of oral mucosa disorder including cancer in many parts of India, particularly in Uttar Pradesh, Madhya Pradesh and some states in the southern India. Further, we also know that smoking in any part of the world (including India) is responsible to as high as 30-40 per cent of all cancer mortality and lung cancer to the list.

We have found in our National Cancer Registry Programme that the incidence of cancer lung is slowly rising and in males it is the number one cancer that falls among the ten leading sites. We also know that heavy use of alcohol is certainly associated with many cancers of the oral cavity, pharynx, larynx, liver and also the rectum. There is also definite information that alcohol and smoking has a synergetic effect in the development of cancer in many sites and we should not ignore the findings and reports of their close association with cancer and lifestyle. We also plan to describe in this Chapter the sexual behaviour that has received greater attention in recent years and the link between cancer of the cervix and sexual habits. Although this is generally very sensitive issue to discuss and even to discuss the relationship of HPV (Human Pappiloma Virus) with high risk of cancer of the cervix. This is proved beyond doubt that HPV plays an important role as a causative factor. A new vaccine against HPV is under investigation and we may start using the same in India very shortly.

Skin Cancer has a definite relationship with solar radiation and is the primary factor in all types of cancers of the skin in white people. Individuals with fair skin are relatively at risk in developing skin cancer. In India, of course, incidence of skin cancer is very low because of the protective phenomenon of the presence of melalin in our skin. However, in the mountainous areas the skin cancer is seen in the population.

There are several other factors which have been described from time to time about the lifestyles and cancer which also need discussion for the benefit of health professionals since it has been found that almost more than 50 per cent of cancers occur due to our lifestyles, peculiar habits.

These can be prevented by our chance in the lifestyle and improvements in our diet intake. This can be a great service to the people and a great opportunity for the medical professionals to prevent cancer in their surroundings.

The Chapter also targets the primary health physicians particularly general physicians who are directly in touch with the population for the health care delivery. They can impart education and awareness to the people that cancer is also a preventable disease and if all-out efforts are made to modify lifestyles and habits we can prevent the disease. A fair amount of success has been achieved in the United States and Europe where some of the prevalent cancers, which occupy a high per cent in the developing countries, have been prevented by concerted efforts of medical professionals and health care workers and by non-governmental organisations.

There are several ways to present and describe the occurrence of cancer in people and its direct and indirect relationship with lifestyles of a population in general and peculiar habits of individuals such as use of irritants which are known to be carcinogens. There are also proven evidence and descriptions that over-nutrition with fat protein and under-nutrition of certain vitamins are linked to the high occurrence of cancer. Considering all these aspects we can divide this Chapter with particular reference to Anatomy and Physiology where the cancer occurrence is high in Indian sub-content.

MOUTH CANCER (ORAL CANCER)

The incidence of oral cancer occupies almost 25 per cent of the total cancers in India and it is found that out of these almost 50 per cent occur in buccal mucousa. The studies show that chewing of tobacco alone or a mixture which is better known as Quid is directly related to the incidence to the consumption of tobacco and the time period the tobacco is kept in the oral cavity particularly in the buccal poach and adjacent areas. It is a fact which we must see with concern that the use of tobacco and its allied substances like pan masala is increasing among the young population including the teenagers and this poses a danger to further increase in the incidence of oral cancer in future. There are several studios in our country including the one wherein the author of this Chapter was involved in the early years of the 60s and 70s with the habit of particular tobacco chewing and constantly holding up of tobacco at the site (buccal mucousa) has direct relationship of occurrence of cancer in the people. This certainly indicates that tobacco components are carcinogenic and some of the components in the form of flouride and other ingredients are higher in chewing tobacco which are harmful and produce cancer. There are also studies which suggest that nitroso-nornecotine (NNN) has been identified as an agent in chewing tobacco that produced an effect on the mucousa of the oral cavity. The other factors found to be associated with oral cancer are under-nutrition particularly vitamins A and C, poor oral hygiene and dental care which are known to produce harmful effects in the oral mucousa. Smoking is also known to affect and has synergetic effects in tobacco chewers in the production of cancer. The use of alcohol is known to be causative factor and can produce harmful effects especially in patients who have the habit of chewing tobacco.

CANCER BREAST

Cancer Breast is a major medical problem with significant burden on the public health network and society. Breast cancer is most common in women in developed countries particularly the Western countries and accounts for almost 30 per cent of all cancers in women. In India, the incidence is 16-20 per cent and however the incidence is slowly rising in urban population which is an alarming situation since this can be on the leading causes of death in women at the prime age of 35-45 years. It is estimated by several studies that the cumulative life time risk of developing breast cancer is almost 10-12 per cent. The average healthy women between the age of 45-50 years have a 5 per cent risk of developing breast cancer. It should be realised that the incidence of breast cancer has been rising slowly in the past several decades and is becoming one of the leading sites in some of the metropolitan cities like Bombay and Delhi and certainly has overtaken carcinoma cervix which was one of the leading sites according to the statistics from population and hospital-based Cancer Registries in India. This is one of the cancers which has direct link with lifestyle and several risk factors have been associated with its development. It has been found that it is related to women with their economic status where the food intake with high fat and protein diet is relatively high, using contraceptives, early monarchy and late menopauses, and women who have developed modern culture especially in breast feeding and interrupted pregnancies. The hormone intake particularly HRT (Hormone Replacement Therapy) in post-menopausal women has direct effect in breast cancer. Delayed full term pregnancy beyond the age of 30 as well as less number of children and even nulliparity have been labelled as risk factors. It is important that additional studies are required to determine whether these factors especially decreased parity or increased age at the first child birth as well as use of contraceptives have direct link with the occurrence of breast cancer. It has been seen that the use of post-menopausal hormone therapy could be a contributing factor in the development of breast cancer. On the contrary, this may precipitate the growth of silent tumours when women starts HRT for menopausal syndrome. (This can be one of the factors where cancer can be diagnosed at an early stage). However, a study is needed in this direction. We are not discussing the family history and hereditary relationship of breast cancer (as this Chapter deals primarily with lifestyles) which certainly is one of the important factors and should be kept in mind that 5-10 per cent of all breast cancers are due directly to inhereditary factors.

In 2010, it is estimated that newly diagnosed cancers in India will surpass the figure one million and cancer deaths will be more than half a million per year in this country as well. These figures show a steady rise in the occurrence of cancer throughout the country. The improvement in diagnosis and awareness among our population about the availability of modern treatment facilities will diagnose more and more cancers. A time has come when the oncologists who are involved in diagnosis and treatment of cancer as also development of better treatment facilities should also effectively work on a programme of cancer prevention. This will certainly reduce the steady rise in the incidence of cancer in India. There are several cancers which were prevalent in Western countries (but are still in very high prevalence in India) but have been reduced significantly—particularly the cancers of oral cavity and cancer of cervix. There are many more cancers which can be prevented by changing the lifestyles and improving our health care programme including public health education, food intake and environmental factors.

The present Chapter also describes the knowledge and information on the causes of cancer in India particularly attributed to lifestyles and measures to prevent them. We should clearly understand that cancer is also a preventable disease and by effecting improvement and change of lifestyles we can do justice to our population. We should involve ourselves as medical professionals in general and oncologists in particular in all the areas of cancer control programme—prevention, early detection, diagnosis, treatment and rehabilitation with our understanding of the origins of chronic diseases notably heart diseases and cancer. There have been several studies particularly generated by epidemiologists and they have clearly demonstrated that many individuals are prone to develop cancer purely on the basis of lifestyles and peculiar habits of their own.

There are several epidemiologic studies conducted in the world and very few in India often beginning with the description of the patients who develop cancer. These patients are assessed to uncover demographic characteristics, medical histories, occupations, habits and lifestyles that may cause cancer.

There is a very definite study reported from the United States that incidence of heart diseases has declined in frequency with changes in lifestyles and introduction of physical upkeeping measures for persons at the age of 35-40 years. The incidence and rates of some of the cancers in the United States as well as in European countries have changed substantially during the last two-three decades. This is purely on the improvements in environment and the suggestions to change the lifestyles particularly use of tobacco and improvement in oral hygiene and addition of vitamins, fresh vegetables and fibre in the diet.

Among women the incidence and mortality rates in uterine cancer particularly of cervix have declined significantly primarily due to the preventive measures and avoidance of known causative factors which produce cancer of the cervix, especially poor local hygiene, inadequate care during pregnancy and frequent pregnancies. Cancer of the colon has also fallen although slightly in recent decades especially by changing food habits and other factors which cause chronic constipation.

The available studies and epidemiologic data certainly implicate food and diet as factors in the etiology of cancer particularly of the digestive system and even other sites. Diet alters the risk of tumours. There have been several studies, national and international, which have demonstrated that dietary factors can modify the risk of cancer—especially oesophagus, stomach, colon, rectum, body uterus as well as breast and prostate. Food addictives particularly food colour and flavouring agents like saccharine (for diabetics) and contaminants like aflatoxin, preservatives and even cooking methods have been found to influence the occurrence of cancer. The studies on obesity and cancer have revealed interlinkage between the two due to the effect of high calories, fat and body weight. The common examples are carcinoma of body uterus due to obesity, body weight and hypertension and diabetes. The incidence has risen considerably in Western countries and is also slowly increasing in India.

Some of the studies have clearly shown a definite co-relation between diet—low in fibre, foliate and other constituents and the increased risk for colon cancer. A study conducted clearly demonstrated a significant lower risk of cancer of the oral cavity and stomach with the use of high intake of vitamin A and fresh vegetables. For general population, several studies including those conducted in India advocated that in order to prevent cancer we should have a definite plan in the National Control Programme and through a major public education programme that encourages consumption of a balanced diet with adequate protein and other needed nutrients, particularly vitamins and fibre-content diet. Some of the measures which have been tried in some parts of the world can be summarised as:

1. Reducing calories and alcohol intake.
2. Increase in the consumption of fresh fruits and vegetables.
3. Awareness through public education that tobacco chewing and pan masala are harmful and can produce dreaded diseases like cancer.
4. Prevention of smoking and intake of alcohol.
5. Improvement in oral and local hygiene.

The people should be told about the advantages and disadvantages of food value in their routine through mass public media—both electronic and press. We are very glad that some of the awareness programmes and preventive measures have been duly started by government and non-governmental organisations for the welfare of the people:

(1) *Alcohol*—lots of calories of little nutritional value—you double your cancer risk if you also smoke. Cut down these and try some of the fruits and juices that can help you reduce the cancer risk.

(2) *Diet* rich in vitamin C particularly in bean salad, melon, broccoli and sweet pepper, tomatoes and spinach can help in prevention of several types of cancers.

(3) Vitamin A which is freely available in your food like bantle, potatoes, carrot, certainly helps in the reduction of cancer of oral cavity.

(4) *Fibre*—it is said that if we eat 4-5 grams of cereal with fibre (and the best source is whole wheat) it will reduce the colon cancer.

The important point is to improve your eating habits and take a balanced food.

In an article in the *British Medical Journal* of January 2000, it was brought out that cigarette smoke contains radio-active fumes. It also mentioned that cigarettes reduce one day life by 11 minutes to the smokers. In another article published as early as 1982 in the *New England Journal of Medicine,* it was indicated that cigarettes contain radioactive elements in the form of Polonium-210 and Lead-210. There were also some additional observations that Lead-210 gets absorbed in the linings of lung and goes into the blood circulation in lung and may go into every tissue and cell in the body. It was also mentioned that in 1932 itself hundreds of smokers stopped smoking after reading this single article in the medical journal. This information will certainly persuade at least many smokers who can quit smoking when they are told that there is radioactivity in the smoking as well.

TOBACCO AND CANCER

Tobacco contains compounds that are known to function as tumour initiators, promoters as well as carcinogens. In several studies it is clearly demonstrated that tumour initiators are mutagens and act at the cellular DNA. It is also known that the effects are irreversable. The promoters are chemical compounds that stimulate excessive proliferation following the initial generation of initiators. This produces pre-cancerous and cancerous lesions in the mucosa of the oral cavity.

In several studies conducted *in vitro* in western countries demonstrated the mutagenic effect of tobacco smoking at the cellular level and also inhibition of DNA repair. It has been found that TSNA found in the smoke are potent carcinogens and nitroso nor nicotine (NNN) are the strongest carcinogens proved in the studies. It is also found that the dose of TSNA to which smokers and snuff users are exposed is comparable to that proved as carcinogenic in animals. It is further reported that subcutaneous injection of TSNA causes tumours of the Nasal cavity. Trachia and Lung in hamesters and in the Nasal cavity, Oesophagus, Lung and Liver in mice. It is further reported that tumours of the nasal cavity, lung, liver and oesophagus have been produced in rats by intra-peritonel administration at TSNA. Further, local application of TSNA into the rat's oral cavity produced malignancy in the cheek (buccal mucosa), tongue and hard pallate. The carcinogenic activity of NNN appears to be organ-specfic for the lung regardless of the root of administration in the animal model used in this study.

In a definite study painting on skin of cigarette smoke

contensates consistently produced papilloma and even carcinoma in more than 40 per cent of the mice. Contensates from pipes and cigars have also produced high incidence of tumour in animal bioassay. It is also observed that application of cigarette smoke contensates *in vivo* to xeno-transplanted human bronchial epithellial cells produce invasive tumours.

Several factors strongly potentiate the carcinogenic activity of tobacco whether used as a smoking or as habitual chewer. Synergenestic effects of alcohol have also been observed in many studies of Oral, Laryngial and Oesophagial cancers with high risk of 10-20 per cent for heavy smokers and drinkers in most of the studies. The combined effect of alcohol and tobacco appeared to be multiplicated. The risk associated with a combined exposure was approximately equal to the product of the risk associated with individual exposures.

LUNG CANCER

The incidence of lung cancer, which is one of the great killers in western and developed countries, is also becoming number one disease in India. During the last five decades an increased incidence and mortality of lung cancer have been observed. The information available in the National Cancer Registry Programme reveals that the disease occurs and is one of the leading sites in males. The reasons for the increase have been attributed to:

(1) Higher cigarette consumption per person, (2) Early start of smoking in adolescents, and (3) Increase in air pollution in metropolitan and major cities. Smokers who indulge in large number of cigarette smoking per day are prone to develop lung cancer at a very early stage of their life. The studies conducted at many parts of the world including India conclude that smoking is directly related to the occurrence of lung cancer and also suggest effective awareness campaign against smoking, to be undertaken by government and non-governmental organisations to safeguard people. The statutory warning printed on the cigarette packets is not enough and some more efforts are needed. In recent years the government is planning to insert some picture particularly on chest diseases which would ultimately lead to lung cancer to

frighten and dissuade people from smoking.

Lung cancer is one of the diseases which has attracted attention throughout the world and the planners to take up the challenge for prevention and especially to reduce smoking and effects changes in lifestyles. Several attempts have been made in the past, for the use of special filters which prevent nicotine or such other chemicals into the epithellium of the bronchus as well as a substitute for smoking. However, we have not seen the significant effect of filter as a preventive measure.

It is also alarming to see that the incidence of lung cancer is proportionately rising in female population as well, since they have also started smoking. There is also extensive studies done on passive smokers at home as well as at work places which can effect non-smokers. This is also to be kept in mind that passive smoking is also harmful. Several studies conducted on patients who have undergone at least three medical annual health checkups revealed that smokers have had the highest adjusted death rate from all causes including cancer, heart diseases and other diseases related to blood vessels. In some other studies particularly conducted in the United States, the investigators have suggested and also concluded that quitting smoking has resulted in substantial reduction in coronary artery diseases. The World Health Day which is observed every year has specifically emphasised on the hazards of smoking and its adverse effects on the health, particularly cancer and heart diseases. They really attempt to give enough information to the people to change their lifestyles and smoking behaviour. In India it is a changing scenario in urban and rural areas that they are switching from beedi to cigarette smoking and this is certainly more harmful and will increase the incidence of the disease particularly cancer in future.

Smoking prevention programme aimed at the youth is an essential requirement by the government and non-governmental organisations. A successful programme should be based on social and psychological theories since the studies conducted in some parts of the world showed that 50 per cent or more reduction has been achieved in young adults when they discontinued smoking when they were informed of the hazards of smoking. A programme to catch them at their school age and those just entered the colleges can prove a great success. The health authorities and certainly social organisations should come forward to provide public education and information to all the persons who are young regarding the adverse effects on their health as a consequence of smoking. There is no more important aspect o! this than the health education of our young and to convince them not to start smoking or to quit smoking before it becomes difficult to drop the habit in future. We also believe that this aspect of imparting education and prevention should not be left to the government alone to solve; rather we should work in unison with voluntary organisations and even to take the message to our schools and colleges. We should do concerted efforts to control one of the most pressing health problems which has a bad effect to our people. They firmly believe that reducing smoking will reduce the devastating toll particularly cancer that affects the nation's health and our health infrastructure.

In some of the studies it is shown that there are somewhat higher rates of lung cancer in low socio-economic population than those higher social classes. This may be either that the low socio-economic class smokes more cigarettes or the higher class population smoke cigarettes accompanied with filter. However, it was not a significant difference to prove that filter is a protective phenomenon. In India, however, the lung cancer is seen in middle and higher social strata of the population

The time has come that we must change our lifestyles and understand that magnitude of our health problem associated with smoking with that of lung cancer, chronic lung diseases and coronary heart diseases.

CARCINOMA OESOPHAGUS

Cancer of the oesophagus has one of the very poor survival rates of all cancers, only about 10 per cent of the patients live five years after diagnosis and adequate treatment and it is a great pity that most die within six months following diagnosis. There are several factors related to this dreaded disease which include dietary factors like spices, hot drinks in the form of Kahba (mostly used in Kashmir) and the food stuff containing nitroso-manine (mostly in the pickles and other food staff). In one of the areas in Karnataka, specifically Dharwad district, the incidence is somewhat higher than that of other places due to a special kind of *roti* which is hard and people take it without butter and *ghee* since they cannot afford. Alcohol and smoking are also causative factors and it is observed that the incidence is 4-5 times higher than those in non-smokers. It is also important to know that cancer of the oesophagus has a very special kind of distribution in the world that right from northern Iran to Kashmir to north China the incidence is very high. This may be a factor related to cold climate which forces the people to take hot beverages including alcohol and some kind of ingredients in the food which can be a contributory factor or even an initiator. It is also said that alcohol has a synergetic interaction with food ingredients that increase the risk or carcinoma oesophagus. Smoking can also be labelled as a contributory factor in these regions.

One of the studies demonstrated that the disease can be prevented by changing the lifestyles and food habits and especially change for a milder ingredient in the drink and especially very hot drink is avoided. It has been proved beyond doubt that thermal component is an important factor in producing carcinoma oesophagus. It is also proved that use of alcohol in combination with thermal trauma a synergetically increases the risk even greater for cancer oesophagus. There is also evidence that nutritional factors especially lack of vitamins, use of dry food (without butter and *ghee*) produce some kind of trauma to mucosa and even has a triggering effect in the production of carcinoma oesophagus.

In India alone Kashmir valley has the highest incidence of carcinoma oesophagus (including stomach).

CARCINOMA OF STOMACH

Diet and environment are known to be important factors in carcinoma of the stomach. This is associated with chronic atrophic intestinal metaplasia of the gastric mucosa. However, the pathogenesis is known to be a complex one with multiple factors including environment and persistent presence of salt and some kind of infection. Helicobector pylori infection produces chronic atrophic gastratics and in presence of nitrates progresses to metaplasia and dysplasia. It is also shown that the co-factors such as spices and some kind of irritants in the food which contain carcinogens contribute to pre-cancerous lesions which progress towards cancer. It is also shown that low intake of vitamin-C and beta-carotine (a recent study revealed changes in the form of dysplasia in the mucosa of the stomach and even the small bowel.

In Japan where the stomach cancer occupies one of the high incidences following World War II. The study identified its relationship with salty foods especially fish, dry fish, and intake of large amount of rice. However, in Japan during the last two decades the situation is very different in that stomach cancer has come down very significantly. This is all because of the changes in lifestyles and food habits as they are now taking more fresh, green and yellow vegetables and even milk which appear to be protective factors. The other closely linked protective factors can be discussed in terms of improvement in economic status especially the use of more vitamin-C and certainly decrease in the use of high risk food which were prevalent in the past. It is also shown that the immigrants from Japan to the United States carry an excessive risk of stomach cancer. However, in due course of time this has reduced to a great significant level and due to improvement in the lifestyles and chances in the food habits and this is a factor certainly which has reduced the incidence of stomach cancer in the migrant population from Japan to the USA.

In India stomach cancer is one of the dominant and takes the fourth position among the leading ten sites especially in Chennai, Trivandrum and Bangalore as compared to other parts of the country.

CANCER OF UTERINE CERVIX

It is estimated and proved by the National Cancer Registry Programme that almost a hundred thousand women suffer from cancer of the cervix which, in fact, is a preventable disease and has been prevented in the Western and developed countries. The disease occurs in 35-45 years of age in India and this is the most productive period of women and more importantly needed in the family. The mortality is very high in some of the developments in treatment technology since the patients attend hospitals in late stage of the disease. Various epidemiological studies and clinical studies conducted in India and abroad have shown that the disease is associated with low socio-economic strata where the local hygiene is very poor, the number of pregnancies and parity are high and care during pregnancy very poor and unhygienic. In recent years, human papilloma virus (HPV 16 and 18) is known to produce cancer of cervix and is closely related with high incidence. This is also known as sexually transmitted disease and has close relationship with lifestyles, low socio-economic environment and poor localisation. There are several studies suggesting simple measures like Pap smear examination and treatment of pre-cancerous lesion which is also known as CIN (Carcinoma Intra-epithellial Neoplasia) and can save previous lives. Simple examinations like Colposcopy and Pap smear are most useful screening procedure in women who are prone to develop cervix cancer. This can be one of the cancer control measures in prevention in populations where the incidence is high? A simple change in the lifestyle with low parity and improvement in local hygiene and certainly the diagnosis of pre-invasive cancer particularly dysoplasia can prevent invasive cancer significant level and save our energy and resources for treatment of such a large number of patients, attending our hospitals in advanced stages.

There can be little doubt that the next few decades will see profound chances in the composition and lifestyles of our population in India. These changes will necessitate alterations and changes in all the aspects of our habits and the health-care delivery system for our people. We must also understand that one of the important changes that will become apparent in our population is an increase in the number of aged people since the average life expectancy is increasing and this is very closely associated with cancer. The effect of the changing age distribution will certainly be felt more strongly in the years to come and will give a major impact, negative as well as positive, on the elderly individuals with cancer.

We should also take into account the role of professionals more and more as they are the main actors who will deal with the changing health scenario and many more health problems of our people. All government, non-governmental and health care professionals should join together and take necessary steps to understand the culture and lifestyles and knowledge about health and health practices. Health Education should form a part of our daily practice and should commence right from the school level. We should also devise some of the visual health educational materials and media messages so that we disseminate information about the occurrence of cancer and its relationship with food habits, use of irritants in the form of tobacco smoking, alcohol consumption, poor nutrition and absence of a balanced diet. The author has often felt frustration by the inaccessibility to information and education for the poor belonging to poor socio-economic strata. All-out efforts should be made to extend all health-care measures for primary prevention of cancer and effecting improvement in their lifestyles. It is a well-known fact that the irritants and other ingredients described as causative factors are almost always contained in their lifestyles and they are also exposed to other factors which have been described in this Chapter and there are prone to develop cancer. A policy is to be defined whereby these population at risk will also be covered. We know it for certain that 50 per cent cancer occurs due to our own lifestyles and use of tobacco and malnutrition. We should therefore see that they get equal opportunities for effecting changes in their lifestyles and habits. It is also necessary that we take the Primary Health Care and the grassroots health care workers into the system so that they are given the responsibility for disseminating the information to the people. They are the professionals who can be used more aggressively in primary and secondary prevention of cancer.

TEN WAYS TO LEAD A HEALTHY LIFE

CHOOSE LIFE, NOT TOBACCO—That should be our motto.

1. Stop smoking.
2. Stop chewing of tobacco and pan masala.
3. Maintain a balanced diet with high fibre.
4. Improve our environment with less pollution.
5. Impart education at the school-level for better hygiene and health needs.
6. Better control of menopausal syndrome in women.
7. Better care during pregnancy.
8. Careful use of contraceptives and hormone replacement therapy.
9. Always be aware of the seven warming signals for cancer.
10. Regular dental and health checkups.

3

CANCER-FREE JOURNEY IN THE MENOPAUSAL ZONE: PAP TEST IS THE PASSPORT

I. INTRODUCTION

A woman's chances of developing cancer uterus increase as she matures. About 95 percent of women with this cancer are 40 years old or older. Especially at risk are women who take estrogen, are post-menopausal, are obese, or have a history of breast cancer or of high blood pressure. The deadliest gynaecologic cancer attacks the ovaries. While a woman is most likely to survive ovarian cancer if it is found early and treated before it has spread outside the ovary, the disease usually has no symptoms. Only 25 percent of ovarian cancers are diagnosed at this early stage. Now many people know that women with two or more close relatives who have had ovarian or breast cancer may be at high risk for developing ovarian cancer. Current research in reducing the risk of ovarian cancer has been promising. One study demonstrated that oral contraceptive pills, in particular those containing the hormone progestin, can cut the risk of ovarian cancer by 50 percent. One of the most preventable and treatable types of cancer is cervical cancer. New screening methods to detect the cancer at its earliest and most treatable stage have significantly reduced the number of deaths from the disease in this country. To help prevent cervical cancer, researchers are focused on the sexually transmitted disease human papillomavirus (HPV), which appears to increase a woman's risk for cervical cancer. Currently, one topic under investigation is the role that HPV plays in blood vessel formation, which is essential for the development of cervical cancer. To detect and to help prevent a gynecologic cancer, women need to have a regular Pap smear test and pelvic exam beginning at age 18 or when they become sexually active. The Pap test can detect HPV infection and pre-cancers of the cervix. During a pelvic exam, the doctor will check the ovaries and uterus for any abnormalities in size or shape. Even women who have had their uterus removed and those past menopause still need to have regular Pap tests, to ensure their best health. We shall concentrate on cancer cervix in this write up.

Cervical cancer is the commonest cancer in the female, in the menopausal zone, in India. While early marriage, poor sexual hygiene and growing extra-marital and pre-marital contacts, multiple sexual partners make the occurrence of this cancer common; fortunately this can be detected with a simple test, even before it takes its foothold firmly in the genitals of the victim. The test is called Pap test, which is easy to perform, and is painless and inexpensive. This test has to be performed regularly every year in all females, who are sexually active at or after the age of 18 years. However, new guidelines say that it can be postponed till 21 years, and instead of annual test it can be done every 2-3 years, if everything else is normal. Remember that though this cancer is usually investigated and generally found in the menopausal zone, where the history is suggestive of early, excessive and varied sexual activity and or smoking/drug abuse, etc. must be examined and investigated properly, in the young age. For that matter one is never too young to ignore Pap smear and other tests, if the conditions are suggestive.

Women who have had a hysterectomy do not need Pap smears unless the hysterectomy was performed for cancer or pre-cancerous conditions. Continue Pap smear screenings for cervical cancer until they are 70 years old. It's important to note that more than **50 percent of diagnosed cases of cervical cancer occur in women who have never had a Pap smear**. Another 10 percent of diagnosed cases of cervical cancer occur in women who have not had a Pap smear in the last five years.

2. WHAT IS PAP SMEAR?

Pap smear is a simple test, which any gynecologist can perform. During a PAP smear some cells are scraped or brushed-off the cervix, and prepared on a slide that is examined under a microscope. The purpose of the Pap test is to detect changes that may lead to cervical cancer long before cancer develops. Pre-cancer of the cervix is easily treated, and almost always prevents cancer from developing. One may see one of the following in the test: either it will be reported as normal, suspicious, pre-cancerous or invasive cancer. Somewhere on the cervix the two cell types, squamous cells and columnar cells meet and **it is in this transformation zone that growth of cancer cells generally occur.**

After the smear has been taken and sent to a laboratory for testing, its report will arrive in due course. The report will be labeled either as normal or abnormal. In case of normal report no further action is required and the person can get it repeated after 1-2 years as per advice and circumstances. An abnormal Pap smear does not necessarily mean that cancer cells were found during the examination. There are many causes for abnormal Pap smear results. Your doctor will evaluate the results to determine if further testing is necessary. A repeat Pap smear may be necessary if you had an infection at the time of the test or if there were not enough cells collected during the test.

The Pap test is a simple, painless test to detect abnormal cells in and around the cervix. A woman should have this test when she is not menstruating; the best time is between 10 and 20 days after the first day of her menstrual period. For about 2 days before a Pap test, she should avoid douching or using spermicidal foams, creams, or jellies or vaginal medicines (except as directed by a physician), which may wash away or hide any abnormal cells.

Since decreased levels of the female hormone estrogen also can influence Pap smear results, menopausal women may need to take estrogen before they repeat the test or perform colostomy examination. Colposcopy is an examination of the cervix and the walls of the vagina, through a speculum. Your doctor looks through a magnifying instrument called a colposcope to detect cervical problems. Colposcopy is always necessary immediately after an abnormal Pap smear has been found. In fact, it will be better if colposcopy is made a part of the routine examination of the cervix, at least in suspicious/ higher than normal risk cases. While waiting to perform another Pap smear test, one should keep an eye on the development of certain symptoms. Pre-cancerous conditions of the cervix seldom cause symptoms. When cancer is present in the cervix, the most common symptom is abnormal bleeding. Bleeding may start and stop between regular menstrual periods, or it may occur after sexual intercourse. Abnormal vaginal discharge is another symptom. Pain is NOT an early warning sign of the disease. But be sure to see your doctor if any of these symptoms arises and esp. if these last longer than 2 weeks.

Don't Skip Important Yearly Examinations that may Save your Life!

As said elsewhere cervical cancer is quite curable when detected early. All women are at risk, some more than the other. Single most important thing is yearly check-up. Early detection and adequate treatment means a difference between life and death. It should begin as soon as woman becomes sexually active. So yearly examination is necessary for a girl in teens onwards to all women well past 50 or later. It is not uncommon to find pre-cancerous cells in young women, but these can be removed successfully.

3. WHAT IS CANCER OF THE CERVIX?

Cancer of the cervix (cervical cancer) is the leading cause of cancer amongst women in India. It is caused by the uncontrolled growth of cells in the cervix. The cervix is the narrowed lower portion of a woman's uterus. Shaped like a cone, it connects the upper portion of the uterus to the vagina and is the "gateway" of the birth canal. Cervical cancer begins slowly, with pre-cancerous changes in the cells lining the inside or outside of the cervix; these changes are generally termed "atypical cells." If left untreated, these atypical cells may go on to a full blown, invasive cancer. Most cases are the result of an infection. About 80-90% of cervical cancers are squamous cell carcinomas, occurring in the flat squamous cells that cover the outside of the cervix. Some other cases are adenocarcinomas, rising from mucus-producing gland cells of the inner side (the opening of the cervix inwards). A few cervical cancers are mixtures of both types.

With early detection, cervical cancer is usually easily treatable. Left unchecked, however, it is almost always fatal. Given time, the cervical cancer can spread (metastasize) to rest of the uterus, the bladder, the rectum, and the abdominal wall. Eventually, it reaches the pelvic lymph nodes and metastasizes. Cervical cancer cells can then invade other organs throughout the body. Invasive cervical cancer is a very common disease in India, since the Pap screening program is not being successfully carried out in this country. In advanced countries with the introduction of the *Papanicolaou (Pap) smear*, a screening tool that allows the detection of cancerous and pre-cancerous changes in the cervix, rates of cervical cancer have dropped by as much as 70%. In developing nations without screening programs, however, cervical cancer is still a very serious concern. Cervical cancer continues to be the second most common type of cancer in women worldwide and number one in India.

4. LIFESTYLE FACTORS

Many persons live in a dangerous lifestyle regarding their habits of food, exercise, entertainment, procreation, sexual relations, etc. They prefer to violate the norms with impunity on the one hand and believe in indulging uncalled for adventurism on the other. With the result they fall pray to serious ailments. Even at this stage they continue to defy the advice of their doctors and other well informed and well meaning friends. Doctors have identified certain risk factors that increase the chance that cells in the cervix will become abnormal or cancerous. Initiation of sexual intercourse before age 18, many sexual partners, early age of marriage, first pregnancy at an early age, four or more number of pregnancies and women with poor personal hygiene, have an increased risk of cervical cancer. Women who have had many sexual partners or whose partners have had many sexual partners may have an increased risk of cervical cancer at least in part because they are more likely to get a sexually transmitted virus. Sexuality is the hottest topic, which has deeply permeated in the minds and bodies of our youth and in others who have crossed the barriers of youthhood long ago. The present generation has come to understand that promiscuity is the peak of enjoyment, without considering the dangers and risks involved. No surprise that 25% of this category of playboys and playgirls are already infected with AIDS and many more with other sexually transmitted diseases (STDs) and viral infections. Scientists believe that some of these viruses may cause the growth of abnormal cells in the cervix and may play a role in cancer development. In several studies co-relation of early sexual activity and contact with multiple partners has been uniformly established. Those who smoke or indulge in any other kind of drug abuse are also more prone to suffer. Though such cancers are far more common in the menopausal zone, early sexual activity and co-habitation with several partners can cause this cancer very early, may be in late teens or early twenties. Though nicotine or other toxic substances themselves are not carcinogenic to the cervix, these do lower the immunity of the body systems and predispose to increased infections and cell changes, leading to cancerous change. Those indulging in substances of abuse also expose themselves to abuse of their bodies. After breast cancer, cervical cancer is the second most common type of cancer in women worldwide but is the commonest cancer among Indian women. This is related to their faulty lifestyle. This also related to their attitude of negligence and procrastination in the matter of early and regular Pap test and other check-ups. Most women with cervical cancer experience a long asymptomatic period before the disease becomes clinically evident. Therefore, early recognition of abnormal cytologic changes through regular screening may prevent progression from pre-invasive to invasive disease. Identifying women at risk for developing invasive cervical cancer enables physicians to appropriately select patients who require continual screening rather than annual screening. Women who are at risk for developing cellular abnormalities include those who smoke and those with a history of sexually transmitted diseases, human papillomavirus (HPV) infection, low socio-economic status, two or more lifetime sexual partners or immunosuppression. The latter factors cause frequent exposure to potential carcinogens, and their requisite presence supports the hypothesis that cervical cancer is a sexually transmitted disease.

5. HOW CAN CANCER OF THE CERVIX BE DETECTED EARLY?

Since it is the early detection that is important to save life or lead a good quality of life and late detection does not help at all, our emphasis is on early detection of symptoms by the patient. Common symptoms of cancer cervix are: Bleeding after sexual intercourse, Bleeding in between menses or post-menopausal bleeding, Excessive white discharge (leucorrhoea), foul odor from the genitals, pain after intercourse, etc. The lady who develops any of these symptoms should report to her gynecologist without any delay. When she visits her doctor with the problem, the doctor first listens to her complaints in detail and then examines her. In a pelvic exam, the doctor checks the uterus, vagina, ovaries, fallopian tubes, bladder and rectum. The doctor feels these organs with her gloved fingers for any abnormality in their shape or size. After this an instrument called speculum is inserted into the vagina. This holds the walls of the vagina apart so that the doctor can see the upper part of the vagina and the cervix. The doctor may then recommend certain tests such as Pap smears, colposcopy, biopsy, dilatation and curettage (D&C), fractional curettage, etc. The pelvic examinations and Pap test allow the doctor to detect abnormal changes in the cervix. If these examinations show that an infection is present, the doctor treats the infection and then repeats the Pap test at a later time. If the examinations or Pap test suggests something other than an infection, the doctor may do other tests to find out what the problem is. The Pap smear test is an easy way to detect early changes in cells of the cervix, the lower end of the uterus or womb. A Pap smear is taken during an internal examination of the vagina. A speculum is inserted into the vagina and some cells are then taken from the cervix using a small spatula and the material is smeared on a glass slide and sent to a medical laboratory to be checked for abnormality. It is important that all women have a Pap smear test at least every two years or more frequently depending upon their sexual activity and hygiene.

Like Pap smear testing, colposcopy is also widely used method to check the cervix for abnormal areas. These tests may not show for sure whether the abnormal cells are present on the surface of the cervix. In that case, the doctor will remove a larger, cone-shaped sample of tissue. This procedure, called conization or cone biopsy, allows the pathologist to see whether the abnormal cells have invaded tissue beneath the surface of the cervix. Conization also may be used as treatment for a pre-cancerous lesion if the entire abnormal area can be removed.

6. A STITCH IN TIME

If all women had pelvic examinations and Pap tests regularly, most pre-cancerous conditions would be detected and treated before cancer develops. Abnormal Pap smear test does not necessarily mean patient is suffering from cancer, but may indicate a pre-cancerous stage. Scientists believe that some abnormal changes in cells of the cervix are the first step in a series of slow changes that can lead to cancer, years later. Appropriate treatment at this time can prevent development of cancer. The patient then needs to be closely followed. That's why it is recommended to have a Pap smear done every two years. That way, most invasive cancers could be prevented. Any invasive cancer that does occur would likely be found at an early, curable stage. So if preventive steps are taken early a serious and life threatening condition can be excluded. So goes the old saying, a stitch in time. Besides prevention of large-scale morbidity and early deaths, this effort will save a lot of money of the sufferers and their families and thus provide economic benefits to the nation as well.

7. SPECIAL TESTS

Besides Pap smear test some other tests may also be valuable to establish the diagnosis and to find out the extent of involvement. Human Pappiloma virus (HPV) test is one such test, which is of tremendous value. HPV testing and typing is available and has been getting a lot of press publicity recently. Determining the presence and strain of HPV in women who have abnormal Pap smears may offer doctors additional information about their patients' risk of developing cervical cancer. However, more research is needed to understand the relationship between HPV and cervical cancer. Although there is a demonstrated link between some strains of HPV and an increased risk of cervical cancer, most women who are infected with HPV do not develop cervical cancer, and many women who do have cervical cancer do not have HPV. It is thought that there may be other factors involved, and HPV testing may eventually prove most useful as an adjunct test to the Pap smear. Similarly, use of Colposcopy; as a follow-up test that involves putting a vinegar-like solution on the cervix and then using a magnifying instrument to look closely at the cervix and checking for abnormal areas. A Schiller test may also be done, in which iodine is placed on the cervix, causing normal cells to turn brown and abnormal cells to show up as white or yellow. A biopsy and microscopic evaluation is the only way to tell for sure whether abnormal cells are cancerous, pre-cancerous, or reactive for some other reason.

Testing for the human papilloma virus (HPV) can accurately identify many pre-cancerous changes in the cervix and may be a useful screening tool in some populations. Some studies have shown that certain types of HPVs cause most cervical cancers, raising the possibility that testing for these HPV types may be one way to screen for the disease. However, there has been uncertainty about how reliable and accurate HPV testing would be. The purpose of one study was to provide data on how HPV testing would perform as a screening tool in a population at high risk for cervical cancer. Women in the study were also screened using other methods, including the conventional Pap test. The test accurately detected a high proportion of the pre-cancerous, high-grade lesions as well as all cases of cervical cancer in this population. 89 percent of the women without high-grade lesions or cancer were accurately classified as negative. Compared to conventional Pap testing, in which cervical cells are examined with a microscope, the HPV test was more sensitive but less specific. The incidence of cervical cancer has fallen considerably in those countries of the world, where intensive screening programs are in place. Since the advent and widespread use of screening Papanicolaou (Pap) smears, which detect asymptomatic pre-invasive lesions at the earliest stages, the incidence of cervical cancer has dramatically decreased from 32 cases per 100,000 women in the 1940s to 8.3 cases per 100,000 women in the 1980s. However, in many parts of the developing world, cervical cancer continues to cause significant morbidity and mortality, India being the leader.

8. HPV AND CANCER CERVIX HAS A CLOSE LINK

Evidence suggests a causal link between HPV infection and cervical neoplasia. This link is strongest for certain HPV types, particularly types 16 and 18. In a prospective study of 297 women with HPV type 18 and cervical cancer, the relative risk of death was 4.4 times greater. Other sub-types, specifically type 16, are also associated with cervical cancer. Other factors, such as smoking, nutrition, coexisting sexually transmitted diseases and genetics, may play a role in a person's susceptibility to HPV sub-types. The presence of high-risk HPV sub-types is associated with a substantial risk of cancer.

Patients with a history of immunosuppression, including human immunodeficiency virus (HIV) infection, require aggressive management, since in these patients; cervical disease follows a more severe and prolonged course. Patients with immunosuppression must deal with persistent infection and the threat of progression to invasive disease. Doctors advise all HIV-positive women to receive semi-annual screening with a Pap smear during the first year after diagnosis. If no cytologic abnormalities are detected, annual screening is recommended thereafter. Immediate colposcopic examination with colposcopic-directed biopsy is warranted if any cytologic abnormalities are found, including atypical cells of undetermined significance.

Cervical neoplasia represents a spectrum of disease that most commonly affects women during their 40s and 50s. The earliest pre-invasive changes, which are squamous intraepithelial lesions, are asymptomatic and usually diagnosed by Pap smear. The intraepithelial neoplasia (mild, moderate or severe) is limited to the cervical epithelium. As invasion occurs, the neoplastic cells penetrate the underlying basement membrane and invade the stroma with the potential for widespread dissemination.

9. SCREENING OF THE CELLS FROM CERVIX, THE PAP TEST ET AL

Since its introduction in the 1940s, the Pap smear has been the standard method of screening of the cervix. Although the false-negative rate of screening Pap smears in the general population reportedly has been as high as 20 to 45 percent, annual screening could lower that rate. Doctors recommend that all women receive screening Pap smears at the onset of sexual activity or at 18 years of age, because strong evidence supports the theory that routine screening with Pap smears will lower the rate of cervical cancer. Once three normal annual Pap smears are documented, the interval for continued surveillance with screening Pap smears might be lengthened at the discretion of the physician and the patient. Inadequately screened populations, such as women more than 65 years of age, Hispanic and African-American women and indigent women, account for 25 percent of the cases of cervical cancer and 41 percent of deaths resulting from the disease. Sixty percent of women who are diagnosed with invasive cervical cancer have not had a Pap smear in the past five years. Women who present for medical care should have initial screening, as well as ongoing surveillance, for the presence of cervical neoplasia.

Pap smears that suggest invasive disease require further evaluation by colposcopy, colposcopic-directed biopsy and endocervical curettage. Colposcopy offers direct visualization of the cervix with an opportunity to biopsy sites of abnormality. Although colposcopy requires additional training to properly differentiate between normal and abnormal epithelium and additional expense to set-up the proper equipment to perform the procedure, family physicians can and must perform the procedure as a part of their outpatient practice.

10. NEW TECHNIQUES TO STUDY CELLS FROM CERVIX: REDUCE FALSE RESULTS

In the past few years, researchers have introduced several new technologies that attempt to increase the sensitivity and decrease the false-negative rate of the conventional screening methods. The U.S. Food and Drug Administration presently label two automated rescreening devices: the AutoPap 300 QC (NeoPath, Redmond, Wash.) and the PapNet (Neuromedical Systems, Suffern, N.Y.). Both are intended to identify possible false-negative results in previously manually screened Pap smears. Auto Pap is set to select 10 percent of the most abnormal Pap smears. This 10 percent, which originally read as normal but are most likely abnormal, are manually rescreened. Pap Net rescreens normal slides, and 128 of the most likely abnormal cells are then manually rescreened by the original laboratory. These services are yet to be introduced in this country.

Another method, called fluid-based cytology, uses a sample of cervical cells that are placed in a fluid media and filtered of blood, mucus and inflammatory cells. A monolayer of cells is then placed on the glass slide for staining and manual screening. This technology aims to decrease false-negative results by optimizing the collection and preparation of cervical cells. Once the diagnosis of invasive cervical cancer is established confidently by histology, the disease is clinically staged, which involves assessment of the degree of dissemination. This assessment allows for consideration of the appropriate treatment options. Pre-treatment evaluation includes taking a thorough history and conducting a physical examination. Particular emphasis should be placed on the pelvic examination, because cervical cancer is often locally destructive before it is metastatic. A rectovaginal examination is important to identify nodules or masses that indicate the possibility of locally invasive disease.

Other Tests

Selective use of chest radiography, intravenous pyelography, cystoscopy, gastrointestinal endoscopy (i.e., flexible sigmoidoscopy), lymphangiography, computed tomography (CT) or magnetic resonance imaging (MRI) of the pelvis and abdomen may be useful in appraising the degree of metastatic disease. Assessment of renal function is vital to the staging of cervical cancer. The presence of unilateral or bilateral ureteral obstruction with azotemia often heralds metastatic disease and heralds a poorer prognosis. Early invasive tumors have a low risk of metastases, if detected early the prognosis is good. Five-year survival exceeds 95 percent with appropriate treatment. Recommended therapy is simple hysterectomy without pelvic lymph node dissection. Adequate cone biopsy with close follow-up is an option in women who wish to preserve their fertility and understand the potential risk of progression.

Radiotherapy involves intracavitary (placement in the vaginal fornices and uterine cavity) and external beam radiation for the treatment of pelvic nodes. Pelvic radiotherapy may also be used when a tumor is found at the margins of the radical hysterectomy specimen or in the pelvic lymph nodes, because it can decrease local recurrence. The presence of lymph node metastasis dramatically decreases survival.

11. HOW CAN CANCER OF THE CERVIX BE TREATED?

Treatment depends on a number of factors, age, location and size of the tumor, including the stage of the disease and the general health of the patient. If cancer is found, it will then be "staged." Staging is a careful and thorough examination and classification of how far the cancer has spread and what body organs are involved. Stages range from Stage 0 (the cancer is found only in the cells covering the cervix) to Stage IV-B (the cancer has spread to other areas of the body, such as the lungs). Staging is a very important part of the diagnostic process for the surgeon-gynecologist to plan treatment options and patient prognosis depends in large part on the stage of the cancer. Thus, staging is a careful attempt to find out whether the cancer has spread and, if so, what parts of the body are affected. Many different treatments and combination of treatments are used to treat cancer of the cervix. The three common modes of cancer treatment are surgery, radiation therapy and chemotherapy. Radiation therapy is the mainstay in the treatment of the cancer of the cervix. It involves subjecting the cancer-bearing region to radiation. Ionizing radiation damages or destroys the cancer cells and prevents them from growing and multiplying. Normally the treatment is divided over a period of one month, during which fixed doses of radiation are delivered each day. Radiation affects both normal as well as abnormal tissues while ensuring sustained tumor destruction. Usually most of the radiation treatment is given as an out-patient procedure. Radiotherapy treatment in itself is painless just like an X-ray, and may take anything from a few seconds to several minutes.

The different radiation therapies involve delivering radiation either from close quarters or from a distance. Radiation therapy where the source of radiation is close to the tumor is referred to as **'Brachytherapy'**. Where the radiation source is located away from the tumor is referred to as **'Teletherapy'**. Brachytherapy is mostly delivered by directly implanting radioactive wires or seeds into the tumor, while Teletherapy is given by using fixed machines. **Surgery** is one of the commonly used modes of cancer treatment, wherein the surgeon removes a localized tumor. **Chemotherapy** is treatment of cancer by drugs. Cancer chemotherapy employs cytotoxic drugs capable of arresting fast cellular growth. Chemotherapy also affects other fast growing and dividing normal cells in the body. The treatment is given in cyclic form once in 3 to 4 weeks, to allow for adequate recovery of normal tissues and to ensure that cancer cells are killed at the same time. Chemotherapy and Radiation therapy may cause side effects, but most side effects of radiotherapy and chemotherapy are reversible after treatment is over.

12. CANCER CERVIX AND PREGNANCY

Pregnancy does not predispose patients to cervical cancer, nor does it change the course of the disease. The rate of cervical cancer in pregnant patients is similar to that in non-pregnant patients of the same age. In patients with concurrent cervical malignancy and pregnancy, the major dilemma is diagnosis and treatment. Diagnosis begins with colposcopic-directed biopsy followed by confirmatory cone biopsy, which carries increased risks of hemorrhage and poor peri-natal outcome. The treatment is a matter of concern to many patients because of the risk to the fetus of exposure to ionizing radiation. There is no evidence of risk to the fetus if the dose of radiation is less than 5 rads. Using "one shot" intravenous pyelograms and substituting MRI for CT scanning can achieve this dosage level. The recommended treatments for pregnant and non-pregnant patients are the same.

Before 20 weeks of gestation, radical hysterectomy should be performed with the fetus *in situ*; beyond 20 weeks, evacuation of the fetus before surgery is recommended. In patients with a pre-viable fetus, delaying therapy until fetal survival is assured is a reasonable option in early disease but is not recommended in patients with more advanced disease. Delivery should be performed as soon as pulmonary maturity of the fetus is demonstrated, although the route of delivery is highly debated. Most experts advocate cesarean delivery, because recurrence of the disease at the site of episiotomy is possible, and delivery through a cervix with advanced cervical cancer increases the risk for hemorrhage, obstructed labour and infection. Squamous cell cancer antigen and other proteins specific to cervical cancer are currently under investigation. The usefulness of these markers in diagnosis continues to be an area of active investigation.

13. FREQUENTLY ASKED QUESTIONS (FAQs) ABOUT CERVICAL CANCER AND OTHER FEMALE CANCERS

1. Can I get pregnant after treatment of pre-cancerous stage?

The pre-cancerous stage or dysplasia itself shouldn't cause infertility, but treatments to the cervix for cervical dysplasia, such as conization by cold knife, LEEP (loop electrical excision procedure), laser or cryosurgery (freezing), can negatively affect the ability to get pregnant. After a year of trying to get pregnant unsuccessfully, it is recommended that you see a physician for diagnosis of *secondary infertility*. If you have a *cervical factor* causing infertility such as the glands destroyed by past cryotherapy, you may need artificial insemination.

2. How do cervical cells change?

We don't know for sure. Many doctors suspect that viruses play a role and stimulate cervical cells to have more nuclear activity. If left alone over many years, that nuclear activity may turn into malignant invasive growth if it progresses.

3. Is cryotherapy required as treatment?

Probably you had a cervical biopsy that showed early cancer. The Pap is only a screening test and what is actually on the cervix can be more abnormal (more severe) than the Pap smear suggests or less abnormal or the same. But all treatment is based on what the colposcopically directed biopsy shows. Usually there are 3 grades; mild, moderate and severe. If the biopsy is a low-grade squamous intraepithelial lesion consistent with mild dysplasia, then cryotherapy isn't really needed at this point. Most of those lesions will regress to normal on their own over-time. It just needs to be followed with every 3 months Paps, but if it progresses then some treatment would be indicated. If you want to get pregnant in the near future. If you had a good colposcopically directed biopsy in which the physician was confident that the worst appearing area was biopsied and it returned as moderate dysplasia, I would put-off treatment with cryo until after you get pregnant. Just follow-up each 3 months with the doctor to see that it doesn't get worse.

4. What are Atypical squamous cells of undetermined significance?

The condition is not serious and one need not get worried over this big name. In this case the cellular changes seen are thought to be mostly a response to some cervical inflammation or irritation, however, some of the inflammation may be due to the human papilloma virus (HPV). HPV usually goes away on its own after a year or two as your body develops immunity to the virus. There are some strains of the virus that are thought to be more aggressive and if left for a long time, may promote more severe changes called dysplasia and even cancer. That is why the Pap changes need to keep being checked, to make sure they don't get worse over time.

5. If a colposcopy is done, is a biopsy necessary?

Atypical squamous cells of undetermined significance (ASCUS) are usually treated by just repeating the Pap smear in 3-6 months. Colposcopy is usually not done unless there are 2 or 3 ASCUS reports in a row. Colposcopy only allows the doctor to see which area of the cervix is giving the abnormal cells so that a biopsy can be directed to the worst area. The biopsy is the "gold standard". Most of the time it needs to be done although sometimes if you've had previous biopsies that are consistent with colposcopic visualization and that visualization has not worsened, a biopsy can be avoided.

6. There is a higher incidence of ASCUS Pap smears progressing to dysplasia in women over age 50, is it true?

Most of the time (70-85%) ASCUS Pap smears revert to normal on their own over time. Women under age 50 have a higher progression of ASCUS pap smears to dysplasia than do menopausal women, but the rates vary considerably depending upon the population studied and the accuracy of the laboratory used. One study has noted that ASCUS Paps over the age of 50 had a lower incidence of progressing to dysplasia—13% *vs.* 30%. Most studies, however, will quote a lower rate of progression to dysplasia for younger women than 30%. It might be time to ask your physician to treat the cervix with some method to get it to produce normal cells and a normal Pap smear. ASCUS changes and even dysplasia are curable by destroying the cervical surface cells by freezing, cautery, LEEP, laser and any procedure that destroys the abnormal cells and stimulates the body's normal cells to repair the damaged ones.

7. What is Unsatisfactory Pap smear?

There are a number of reasons why a Pap smear may be read as unsatisfactory. These include a thick normal vaginal secretion, but more commonly cervical or vaginal infection will give you inflammation. Also some of the endocervical cells may not have been collected on the slide. Rarely a menstrual period may result in too many blood cells and not enough epithelial cells to assess. Anything that obscures the cytologist being able to see enough of the expected cells will result in a report of unsatisfactory. This is not an abnormal report, just a pain in the bottom because it should be repeated. And yes, the doctor did scrape your cervix, as that is what he/she needs to do to obtain the sample. Keep in mind, however, that the "scraping" is just to pick up cells that have already been sloughed-off of the cervical surface. Scraping does not remove a layer of growing cells on the cervix.

8. Why are a Pap smear and pelvic exam important?

A Pap test and pelvic exam are important parts of a woman's routine health care because they can detect abnormalities that may lead to invasive cancer. These abnormalities can be treated before cancer develops. Most invasive cancers of the cervix can be prevented if women have Pap tests and pelvic exams regularly. Also, as with many types of cancer, cancer of the cervix is more likely to be treated successfully if it is detected early.

9. Who performs a Pap test?

Doctors and other specially trained health care professionals, such as physician assistants, nurse midwives, and nurse practitioners, may perform Pap tests and pelvic exams. These individuals are often called clinicians.

10. How is a Pap test done?

A Pap test is simple, quick, and painless; it can be done

in a doctor's office, a clinic, or a hospital. While a woman lies on an exam table, the clinician inserts a speculum into her vagina to open it. To do the test, a sample of cells is taken from in and around the cervix with a wooden scraper or a small cervical brush or broom. The specimen (or smear) is placed on a glass slide or rinsed in liquid fixative and sent to a laboratory for examination.

11. Who should have Pap test?

Women who are or have been sexually active, or have reached age 18, should have Pap tests and physical exams regularly. Women may want to discuss with their doctor how often to have the test. There is no known upper age at which Pap tests cease to be effective. Older women should continue to have regular physical exams, including pelvic exams and Pap tests. Women who have had consistently normal Pap test results may want to ask the doctor how often they need to have a Pap test.

Women who have had a hysterectomy (surgery to remove the uterus, including the cervix) should talk with their doctor about whether to continue to have regular Pap tests. If the hysterectomy was performed for treatment of a pre-cancerous or cancerous condition, the end of the vaginal canal still needs to be sampled for abnormal changes. If the uterus (including the cervix) was removed because of a non-cancerous condition such as fibroids, routine Pap tests may not be necessary. However, it is still important for a woman to have regular gynecologic examinations as part of her health care.

12. When should the Pap test be done?

A woman should have this test when she is not menstruating; the best time is between 10 and 20 days after the first day of the menstrual period. For about 2 days before a Pap test, she should avoid douching, or using vaginal medicines or spermicidal foams, creams, or jellies (except as directed by a physician). These may wash away or hide abnormal cells.

13. How are the results of a Pap test reported?

The way of reporting Pap test results has sometimes been confusing. The present system will tell whether the cells are normal, inflammatory, atypical, dysplasia or frank invasive. This system of reporting includes an evaluation of specimen adequacy.

14. What do abnormal test results mean?

A physician may simply describe Pap test results to a patient as "abnormal." Cells on the surface of the cervix sometimes appear abnormal but are not cancerous. There are several terms that may be used to describe abnormal results:

- Dysplasia is a term used to describe abnormal cells. Dysplasia is not cancer, although it may develop into very early cancer of the cervix. In dysplasia, cervical cells undergo a series of changes in their appearance. The cells look abnormal under the microscope, but they do not invade nearby healthy tissue. Squamous intraepithelial lesion (SIL) is another term that is used to describe abnormal changes in the cells on the surface of the cervix. The word squamous describes cells, which are thin, flat, and lie, on the outer surface of the cervix. The word "lesion" refers to abnormal tissue. An intraepithelial lesion means that the abnormal cells are present only in the surface layers of the cells. A doctor may describe SIL as being low-grade (early changes in the size, shape, and number of cells) or high-grade (a large number of pre-cancerous cells that look very different from normal cells).
- Cervical intraepithelial neoplasia (CIN) is another term that is sometimes used to describe abnormal cells. Neoplasia means a new abnormal growth of cells. Intraepithelial refers to the surface layers of the cells. The term CIN, along with a number (1 to 3), describes how much of the cervix contains abnormal cells.
- Carcinoma *in situ* describes a pre-invasive cancer

that involves only the surface cells and has not spread into deeper tissues. Cervical cancer, or invasive cervical cancer, occurs when abnormal cells spread deeper into the cervix or to other tissues or organs.

15. What are atypical squamous cells of undetermined significance (ASCUS)?

Abnormalities that do not fulfil the criteria that define SIL, CIN, or dysplasia are termed atypical squamous cells of undetermined significance (ASCUS). A physician often further evaluates persistent abnormal smears.

16. Is the human papillomavirus associated with the development of cervical cancer?

Human papillomaviruses (HPV) are viruses that can cause warts. Some HPVs are sexually transmitted and cause wart-like growths on the genitals. Scientists have identified more than 70 types of HPV; 30 types infect the cervix, and about 15 types are associated with cervical cancer. HPV is a major risk factor for cervical cancer. In fact, nearly all cervical cancers show evidence of HPV. However, not all cases of HPV develop into cervical cancer.

17. Who is at risk for HPV infection?

HPV infection is more common in younger age groups, particularly in women in their late teens and twenties. Because HPV is spread mainly through sexual contact, risk increases with number of sexual partners. Women who become sexually active at a young age, who have multiple sexual partners, and whose sexual partners have other partners are at increased risk. Non-sexual transmission is also possible. The virus often disappears but may remain detectable for years after infection.

18. Does infection with a cancer-associated type of HPV always lead to a pre-cancerous condition or cancer?

No. Most infections appear to go away on their own without causing any kind of abnormality. However, infection with cancer-associated HPV types may increase the risk that mild abnormalities will progress to more severe abnormalities or cervical cancer. With regular follow-up care by trained clinicians, women with pre-cancerous cervical abnormalities should not develop invasive cervical cancer.

19. What are false positive and false negative results?

Unfortunately, there are occasions when Pap test results are not accurate. Although these errors do not occur very often, they can cause anxiety and can affect a woman's health.

A false positive Pap test occurs when a patient is told she has abnormal cells when the cells are actually normal. A false negative Pap test result occurs when a specimen is called normal, but the woman has a lesion. The Food and Drug Administration has recently approved two computerized systems for rescreening of samples to detect abnormal cells from a Pap test. These systems are beginning to be used in laboratories across the country. Rescreening may also be done manually.

20. What is the difference between pre-cancerous conditions and cancer of the cervix?

Cells on the surface of the cervix sometimes appear abnormal but not cancerous. Scientists believe that some abnormal changes in cells on the cervix are the first step in a series of slow changes that can lead to cancer years later. Over the years, doctors have used different terms to refer to abnormal changes in the cells on the surface of the cervix. One term now used is squamous intraepithelial lesion (SIL). Changes in these cells can be divided into two categories:

- Low-grade SIL (LGSIL) refers to early changes in the size, shape and number of cells that form the surface of the cervix. Some low-grade lesions go away on their own. However, with time, others may grow larger or become more abnormal, forming a high-grade lesion. Pre-cancerous low-grade lesions also may be called mild dysplasia or cervical intraepithelial neoplasia 1 [CIN 1 High-grade SIL (HGSIL)] means that the pre-cancerous changes are more severe; they look very different from normal cells. Like low-grade SIL, these pre-cancerous changes involve only cells on the surface of the cervix. HGSIL on a Pap smear may be associated with malignancy of the cervix. Therefore, a proper diagnostic evaluation is necessary. They develop most often in women between the ages of 30 and 40 but can occur at other ages as well. If abnormal cell spread deeper into the cervix or to other tissues or organs, the disease is then called cervical cancer, or invasive cervical cancer. The average age of cervical cancer is 50.

21. How do I read my Pap smear results so that I can understand them?

The following table will help you to better understand your Pap smear results:

Results	*Description*	*Follow-up*
Within Normal Limits	No abnormal cells detected.	Return for pelvic exam and Pap test in one year.
Atypical cells	Some cells show a few changes, or mild atypical. These changes might be due to a type of infection or Human Papilloma Virus (HPV).	There is not one standard management plan for a patient with an ASCUS Pap smear. The appropriate follow-up and testing will depend on the patient's personal history. Nevertheless, appropriate evaluation usually includes a repeat Pap smear and/or colposcopic examination. Sometimes the inflammation is due to an infection or some other irritant and resolves with appropriate treatment.

22. What are the symptoms of cancer of the cervix?

Pre-cancerous changes of the cervix usually do not cause pain. In fact, they generally do not cause any symptoms and are not detected unless a woman has a pelvic exam and a Pap test. Symptoms usually do not appear until abnormal cervical cells become cancerous and invade nearby tissue. Abnormal

Bleeding (bleeding may start and stop between regular menstrual periods). Bleeding after intercourse, douching, or pelvic exam. Menstrual bleeding may last longer and be heavier than usual. Bleeding after menopause may be a symptom of cancer of the cervix increased vaginal discharge. It is important for a woman to contact her doctor if she is having any of these symptoms.

23. How is cancer of the cervix diagnosed?

The pelvic exam and Pap test allow the doctor to detect abnormal changes in the cervix. If these exams show that an infection is present, the doctor treats the infection and then repeats the Pap test at a later time. If the Pap test or exam suggests something other than an infection, the doctor may repeat the Pap test and do other tests to find out what the problem is. The Pap smear is only a screening test and does not give a final diagnosis. A diagnosis and subsequent treatment is based on biopsy results, which are usually obtained after an abnormal Pap smear is discovered. **Colposcopy** is a widely used method to check the cervix for abnormal areas. This procedure is most commonly performed after an abnormal Pap smear. The doctor applies a vinegar-like solution to the cervix and then uses an instrument much like a microscope (called a colposcope) to look closely at the cervix. Schiller Test—The doctor may coat the cervix with an iodine solution. Healthy cells turn brown; abnormal cells turn white or yellow.

These procedures can be done in the doctor's office.

Endocervical Curettage (ECC)—The doctor may want to check inside the opening of the cervix. The doctor uses a curette (a small, spoon-shaped instrument) to scrape tissue from inside the cervical opening. In some other cases the doctor may decide to perform curettage of all the walls of the uterus, called fractional curettage. Conization—Also called Cone Biopsy. This procedure requires either local or general anesthesia and may be done in the doctor's office or in the hospital. This procedure allows for evaluation and treatment of pre-cancerous lesions. The conization also may provide the diagnosis of an invasive cervical cancer lesion. In a few cases, it may not be clear whether an abnormal Pap test or a woman's symptoms are caused by problems in the cervix or in the endometrium (the lining of the uterus). In this situation, the doctor may do dilatation and curettage (D&C). The doctor stretches the cervical opening and uses a curette to scrape tissue from the lining of the uterus as well as from the cervical canal. Like conization, this procedure requires local or general anesthesia and may be done in the hospital.

24. How are pre-cancerous conditions of the cervix treated?

All treatments directed towards neoplastic conditions of the cervix should be based on a biopsy and not a Pap smear alone. Treatment for a pre-cancerous lesion of the cervix depends on a number of factors. These factors include whether the lesion is low or high grade, whether the woman wants to have children in the future, the woman's age and general health, and the preference of the woman and her doctor. A woman with a low-grade lesion may not need further treatment, especially if the abnormal area was completely removed during biopsy, but she should have a Pap test and pelvic exam regularly by a physician with expertise in this area. When a pre-cancerous lesion requires treatment, the doctor may use: Cryosurgery (Freezing), Cauterization Burning (also called diathermy), Laser Surgery—To destroy abnormal area without harming nearby healthy tissue, LEEP—Loop Electro Surgical Excision Procedure Conization—Cone Biopsy.

Treatment for pre-cancerous lesions may cause cramping or other pain, bleeding, or a watery discharge. Occasionally, a hysterectomy is performed to treat pre-cancerous conditions of the cervix. However, the hysterectomy is considered to be unnecessary in the great majority of cases of pre-cancerous conditions of the cervix unless other gynecologic problems co-exist.

25. How is cancer of the cervix treated?

The choice of treatment for cervical cancer depends on the location and the size of the tumor, the stage (extent) of the disease, the woman's age and general health and other factors. Gynecologic oncologists have surgical expertise in the procedures of radical hysterectomy, pelvic and Para-aortic lymphadenectomy, pre-treatment surgical staging procedures, and exenterations for those patients with recurrent cervical cancer. Gynecologic oncologists also work closely with radiation therapists when this is the primary treatment modality. Staging is a careful attempt to find out whether the cancer has spread and, if so, what parts of the body are affected. Blood and urine tests are usually done. The doctor also may do a thorough pelvic exam in the operating room with the patient under anesthesia. During this exam, the doctor may do procedures called cystoscopy and proctosigmoidoscopy. In cystoscopy, the doctor looks inside the bladder with a thin, lighted instrument. Proctosigmoidoscopy is a procedure in which a lighted instrument is used to check the rectum and the lower part of the large intestine. Because cervical cancer may spread to the bladder, rectum, lymph nodes, or lungs, the doctor also may order X-rays or tests to check these areas. For example, the woman may have a series of X-rays of the kidneys and bladder, called an intravenous pyelogram (IVP). The doctor also may check the intestines and rectum using a barium enema. To look for lymph nodes that may be enlarged because they contain cancer cells, they may order a CT scan, a series of X-rays put together by a computer to make detailed pictures of areas inside the body. Other procedures that may be used to check organs inside the body are ultrasonography and MRI.

26. Is a second opinion important?

Before starting treatment, you may wish to have a second opinion to review the diagnosis and treatment plan. A gynecologist is usually in the best position to offer a patient an expert opinion on the diagnosis and management of cervical cancer. A multi-disciplinary meeting where gynecologic oncologists, radiation therapy physicians and gynecologic pathologists along with the attending gynecologists meet to discuss the diagnostic and treatment options for a patient with or suspected to have a malignancy.

27. What can I do to prepare for treatment?

Here are some questions you may ask your doctor before treatment begins: What is the stage (extent) of my disease? What are my treatment choices? Which do you recommend? Why? What are the chances that the treatment will be successful? What are the risks and possible side effects of each treatment? How long will treatment last? Will it affect my normal activities? What is the treatment likely to cost? What is likely to happen without treatment? How often will I need to have check-ups?

When a person is diagnosed with cancer, shock and stress are natural reactions. These feelings may make it difficult for patients to think of everything they want to ask the doctor.

28. What is DES?

DES (diethylstilbestrol) is a synthetic form of estrogen, a female hormone. It was prescribed from the early 1940s until 1971 to help women with certain complications of pregnancy. Use of DES declined in the 1960s after studies showed that it might not be effective in preventing pregnancy complications. Also when given during the first 5 months of a pregnancy, DES can interfere with the development of the reproductive system of the fetus. For this reason, although DES and other estrogens may be prescribed for some medical problems, they are no longer used during pregnancy.

In 1971, DES was linked to an uncommon cancer (called clear cell adenocarcinoma) in a very small number of daughters of women who had used DES during pregnancy. This cancer of the vagina or cervix usually occurs after age 14, with most cases found at age 19 or 20. The upper age limit, if any, for DES-exposed daughters to develop this type of cancer is not known, and some cases have been reported in women in their thirties and forties. The overall risk of an exposed daughter to develop this type of cancer is estimated to be between 1/1000 (0.1%) and 1/10,000 (0.01%). Physicians use a number of terms to describe these abnormal cells, including dysplasia, cervical intraepithelial neoplasia (CIN), and squamous intraepithelial lesions (SIL). These abnormal cells resemble cancer cells in appearance; however, they do not invade nearby healthy tissue as cancer cells do. These abnormal cellular changes usually occur between the ages of 25 and 35 but may appear in exposed women of other ages as well. Although this condition is not cancer, it may develop into cancer if left untreated. DES-exposed daughters should have a yearly Pap smear and pelvic exam to check for abnormal cells.

DES-exposed daughters also may have structural changes in the vagina, uterus, or cervix. Most of these structural changes do not cause medical problems. In addition, they also may have irregular menstruation and an increased risk of miscarriage, tubal (ectopic) pregnancy, infertility, and premature delivery. Women who used DES may have a slightly increased risk of breast cancer. Previous research indicates that the risk of breast cancer in DES-exposed mothers is approximately 30 percent higher than the risk for women who have not been exposed to this drug.

What is required for DES exposed females?

(i) *Pelvic examination*—A physical examination of the reproductive organs. An examination of the rectum also should be done.

(ii) *Palpation*—As part of a pelvic examination, the doctor feels the vagina, uterus, cervix, and ovaries for any lumps. Often palpation provides the only evidence that an abnormal growth is present.

(iii) *Pap test*—A routine cervical Pap test is not adequate for DES-exposed daughters. The cervical Pap test must be supplemented with a special Pap test of the vagina called a "four-quadrant" Pap test, in which cell samples are taken from all sides of the upper vagina.

(iv) *Iodine staining of the cervix and vagina*—An iodine solution is used to temporarily stain the linings of the cervix and vagina to detect adenosis (a non-cancerous but abnormal growth of glandular tissue) or other abnormal tissue.

(v) *Colposcopy*—In colposcopy, a magnifying instrument is used to view the vagina and cervix. Some doctors do not perform colposcopy routinely, but if the Pap test result is not normal, it is very important to check for abnormal tissue.

(vi) *Biopsy*—Small samples of any tissue that appear abnormal on colposcopy are removed and examined under a microscope to see whether cancer cells are present.

(vii) *Breast examinations*—Thus far, DES-exposed daughters have not been shown to have a higher risk of breast cancer than unexposed daughters; however, they should follow the routine screening recommendations for their age group.

29. What is Chemotherapy Fatigue?

The patients of cancer cervix on chemotherapy treatment say they are "bone-tired". Simple things like taking a bath or even eating a full meal are exhausting. Most cancer patients will feel this extreme fatigue for weeks or months. This feeling is considered the No. 1 side effect of cancer and largely is caused by the chemotherapy or radiation necessary to fight the disease. Yet few patients seek or receive treatment for fatigue. Studies suggest that over 75 percent of cancer patients suffer serious fatigue. It limits their ability to work, attend school or perform daily activities. There is a mental toll where patients cannot concentrate, are forgetful or depressed. It even can hinder rigorous cancer therapy. Part of the problem is dispelling the myths that there is no help for fatigue, or that fatigue only could mean the cancer is worsening so patients are scared to mention it. Anemia is a leading culprit, because radiation and many powerful chemotherapy drugs that kill cancer cells also kill blood and bone-marrow cells. Medicines, such as Epogen or Procrit, that boost blood-cell production or blood transfusions may help. Under treated pain is another big cause, limiting patients' sleep. Some new studies suggest mild exercise programs help, because constant rest actually makes patients quickly lose muscle strength, thus worsening fatigue. Tumors can compete for a body's nutrients at the same time that chemotherapy-caused nausea depletes calories and spurs dehydration. There are medicines to minimize nausea, and nutritionists may suggest easier-to-tolerate, high-nutrient meals. Sometimes help can be creative: Put a chair under the shower or a rolling stool in the kitchen to conserve energy. The attending doctor may not fully understand the degree of fatigue and that is frustrating to patients, as is finishing treatment and still being fatigued.

30. What is the importance of Abnormal uterine bleeding and family history of uterine cancer?

I have had abnormal bleeding on/off for the past 3 years. Also I have a family history of uterine cancers, what does it mean?

Three years is a long time to have abnormal uterine bleeding and not have a diagnosis or treatment. Uterine cancer can be endometrial (the lining of the uterus), cervical (abnormal Paps, etc.) or rarely the muscle of the uterus. Did everyone in the family have endometrial cancer (not cervical cancer) that you know of? There are some genetic tendencies toward early endometrial cancer. While usually endometrial biopsies or D&Cs are not done to rule out cancer at ages less than 35 or 40, that only applies to initial presentations of abnormal bleeding. If bleeding persists after attempts at hormonal therapy it still needs to be evaluated, including possibly an endometrial biopsy even at age 25. There are very few drugs or medications known to prevent any cancer but birth control pills have definitely been shown to prevent endometrial cancer if taken over a long period of time.

31. Use of Clomid and risk of ovarian cancer?

There does appear to be an increase in the lifetime risk of ovarian cancer in women who had long-term use of Clomid for ovulation induction.

32. What are symptoms of ovarian cancer?

There are no symptoms at all for early ovarian cancer (Stages I and II), because it is a slow growing process and doesn't cause pain. Advanced cancers have symptoms, however, usually including abdominal fullness and feeling full and not hungry all of the time. Increasing abdominal girth can also be a late sign because of fluid in the abdominal cavity.

33. Abdominal bloating, could it be ovarian cancer?

Abdominal bloating can be a sign of ovarian cancer but it is always very slow in onset (over many months) and rarely causes pain and cramps until very late in the disease. Ovarian cancer is usually a disease of the 50s and 60s. Ovarian cysts, endometriosis, fibroids, adenomyosis and infection would be possible. How frequently are you having to pass urine? Does it burn? Do you get up at night to void? Does pain get worse or better with bowel movement or voiding. Are you on anything for birth control. When was your last pelvic exam? Was it normal?

34. Birth control pills and ovarian cancer prevention, any link?

Longtime pill use (over 10 years) is associated with a decreased incidence of ovarian cancer just as having 5 children is also associated with a decrease. This is probably because the less the ovary is allowed to ovulate, the less it is exposed to cancer causing agents. If that's true (we are not certain it is), then Depoprovera use, nursing your children for long periods of time and any diseases or stress that makes a woman anovulatory would also decrease the lifetime incidence of ovarian cancer.

35. Vaginal bleeding 5 years after cervical cancer therapy, What does it mean?

I know you are concerned about the possible recurrence of cancer as the cause of the bleeding. Since that took place 5 years ago, it is much less likely to be a cancer recurrence than it is a vaginal tear or abrasion. You are right to consider mostly bleeding due to trauma with sexual relations because she has risk factors for atrophic vaginitis. The radiation therapy decreases vaginal and pelvic blood supply which in turn makes the skin lining the vagina quite thin. Actually it can be more of a problem farther away from the time of the actual radiation therapy, i.e., it is a late occurrence complication.

Not taking the estrogen replacement therapy is also a risk factor since she is probably menopausal from the radiation therapy. Frequent sexual relations can thicken the vaginal skin lining and make it resistant to bleeding but when you combine that with a history of radiation therapy, the epithelium (skin) may just be too thin to resist abrasion and then secondary infection. The oncologist may have to do a biopsy and other studies just to be sure there is no cancer recurrence.

36. Are there similarities between colon and ovarian cancer?

Ovarian cancer has been described in association with three autosomal dominant syndromes: familial site-specific ovarian cancer, familial breast and ovarian cancer, and the hereditary non-polyposis colon cancer syndrome. If your sister does not have this type of colon cancer I am not aware of any connection.

37. Numbness 2 years after ovarian cancer surgery, any connection with cancer?

It is possible that the cyst is causing the pain. It may be by direct pressure on the lateral femoral cutaneous nerve but it more likely to be a referred pain because the ovary is innervated by some of the same nerve roots as is the lateral femoral cutaneous nerve.

This is called referred pain because you perceive it from one area when actually it originates in another. Remember also that you can have direct pressure on the nerve from anything in the pelvis. It's unlikely that the new numbness is related to cancer. After an ultrasound and possibly a CAT scan, the next step is to look surgically. There can be adhesions that are causing this.

14. CERVICAL CANCER NEWS AND TRENDS

(a) Herpes, HPV May Spell Cervical Cancer (Health Scout News—06/11/2002)

New research suggests that herpes and another common sexually transmitted virus can be a deadly combination, raising the risk that infected women will develop cervical cancer. The findings seem to explain why some women are more prone to cervical cancer. "We know that HPV (human papillomavirus) causes cancer, but a lot of people have HPV and never get cancer," explains Stephen E. Hawes, an assistant professor of epidemiology at the University of Washington at Seattle and author of a commentary on the new study.

An estimated 13,000 American women fall victim to cervical cancer each year and 4,100 will die, according to the American Cancer Society. However, tests known as Pap smears let many more stop the disease in its tracks before it becomes serious. Deaths from the cancer dropped by 74 percent from 1955 to 1992, after the tests became popular. Scientists think at least 90 percent of cervical cancer cases are caused by HPV, which may be the most common sexually transmitted disease. HPV causes inflammation, which makes the cervix more hospitable to cancerous cells by preventing them from dying naturally, Hawes explains. "This process can take years to develop—20 to 30 years after you have your initial HPV infection," he says.

Some scientists have suspected that herpes could make things worse. An international group of researchers tested that theory by examining medical records from seven countries of 1,263 women with cervical cancer and 1,117 women free of the disease. The findings appear in the *Journal of the National Cancer Institute*. The researchers from the International Agency for Research on Cancer found signs of infection with herpes simplex virus 2 in about 44 percent of the women with cancer, but only in 26 percent of the other women. They also found HPV in nearly 95 percent of the women with cancer, but only in 15 percent of the healthy women. Of all women who were infected with HPV, herpes increased their risk of cervical cancer by two to three times.

Dr. Tom Wright, a pathologist at Columbia University, says the findings confirm those of a 1991 study in Latin America. However, it's still unclear how herpes works to make women more susceptible to cervical cancer since the virus doesn't cause as much dangerous inflammation, he adds. There is hope for the future, however. "The biggest issues right now are the development of vaccines to prevent infection with high-risk types of HPV and new molecular tests to identify those women at greatest risk for developing cervical cancer," he says.

(b) New Technique Tested Against Cervical Cancer (Reuters—04/09/2002)

British scientists have devised a new technique that kills cervical cancer cells without harming healthy ones, which could improve treatment for the deadly disease. The technique, called RNA interference, wipes out the deadly cells by silencing genes in a virus that contributes to the illness.

"Our work has identified a novel agent with major therapeutic potential for the treatment, and possibly also the prevention, of human cervical cancer," Professor Jo Milner, of the University of York, said. Unlike chemotherapy, which has serious side effects because it destroys healthy as well as cancerous cells, RNA interference restores the immune system and only targets the cancerous cells. Cancer develops when something goes wrong during normal cell division and instead of destroying itself; the mutated cell develops uncontrollably and forms a tumor.

Cervical cancer, the second most common cancer in women worldwide, is linked to the human papilloma virus, which attacks two important proteins in the body called p53 and RB. RB controls cell division and p53 kills damaged cells that could become cancerous. Without them mutated cells can multiply uncontrollably. But in laboratory studies using cancer cells from human tumors, Milner and Dr. Ming Jiang found that when they silenced two genes in the virus all the cancer cells died while healthy cells were not harmed. Their research is reported in the *Journal Oncogene*. "As soon as we silenced the viral genes, the infected cancer cells committed suicide," said Milner, adding that the results were "absolutely remarkable."

Cervical cancer affects about 465,000 women worldwide each year and causes 300,000 deaths. If the illness is diagnosed and treated early there is a high survival rate.

(c) More Details on Cervical Cancer Virus Link (Reuters Health—25/07/2002)

Human papillomavirus (HPV) is known to increase cervical cancer risk. Now Dutch researchers have found this risk may be increased 100 times among women harboring a certain strain of the virus. There are more than 100 different types of HPV, including some that cause genital warts. Some of these viruses are sexually transmitted, and some are linked to cancer. It is believed that certain "high-risk" HPV sub-types are the primary cause of cervical cancer. However, HPV infection usually goes away on its own, and most women who get the virus do not develop cervical cancer.

In the study, Dr. Yolanda van der Graaf of the University

Medical Center, Utrecht in the Netherlands and colleagues examined the medical records of 77 women who developed cervical cancer and had submitted Pap smears before being diagnosed with the disease. The researchers went back and tested the Pap smears for signs of HPV and compared the test results from cancer patients to 270 women who did not develop the disease. The average follow-up time between disease-free Pap smear and cancer diagnosis was 5-1/2 years.

Reporting in a recent issue of the *American Journal of Epidemiology*, the investigators found that 71% of women who later developed cervical cancer received earlier Pap smears that showed no sign of cervical cancer, but did contain HPV. In contrast, only 11% of women who never developed cervical cancer had earlier Pap smears that tested positive for HPV. These numbers translate into a 19-fold increased risk of developing cervical cancer for women infected with HPV.

The link between HPV and future risk of cervical cancer was especially strong in women infected with high-risk sub-types of the virus, the report indicates. Women infected with the sub-types 18, 31 or 33 were more than 50 times as likely to develop cervical cancer as uninfected women. Furthermore, those who were infected with the 16 sub-types showed a more than 100-fold increased risk of cancer compared with those who were virus-free, the team found. While many women with HPV eventually clear themselves of the infection, for a minority of women HPV persists. Previous research has shown that women with persistent infections are more likely than others to develop tissue abnormalities that can become cancerous. Indeed, in this study, van der Graaf and colleagues found that 78% of women who later developed cervical cancer had persistent HPV infections. The link between HPV type and cancer has led researchers to consider whether screening women for HPV might act as an early test for cervical cancer. If laboratories are able to pinpoint certain HPV sub-types, as well as the amount of virus present in samples, the authors write, testing for HPV may indeed become useful as a primary screening tool for cervical cancer.

(d) Study finds Pill Increases Cervical Cancer Risk in Some Women (Associated Press—26/03/2002)

Women infected with the common sexually transmitted human papilloma virus could be more likely to develop cervical cancer if they have taken birth control pills for a long time, new research has found. Some gynaecologists believe that contraceptive pills might increase the risk of cervical cancer, but others are doubtful because previous studies have not ruled out the possibility that pill users might simply be more likely to be infected with the human papilloma virus, the main cause of cervical cancer. Experts say the new study, conducted by the International Agency for Research on Cancer, an arm of the World Health Organization, lends support to the view that there is a real connection between birth control pills and cervical cancer.

However, Dr. Jack Cuzick, head of mathematics, statistics and epidemiology at Cancer Research, UK in London, who was not connected with the study, said the findings should be interpreted cautiously because the women were only tested for the human papilloma virus, or HPV, once. "Ideally, they should be positive on two occasions, at least six months apart, before you call them positive," he said.

The human papilloma virus, or HPV causes virtually all cervical cancer. Nearly all sexually active women will be infected by HPV sometime during their lives, but in most cases the immune system quickly eliminates it. The key issue is why, in some cases, the virus is not eliminated. If the infection persists, the chances of cancer increase enormously. "This study suggests that if you've got an HPV infection, oral contraceptives may actually be promoting the rate at which that progresses to cancer," Cuzick said.

The research was to be published on the Web site of *The Lancet Medical Journal.*

The WHO researchers pooled evidence collected in eight earlier studies of 3,769 women from four continents, which were tested for HPV and told the investigators about their use of birth control pills. A total of 1,853 had cervical cancer, while 1,916 did not. As expected, nearly all the women with cancer tested positive for HPV, while hardly any who were cancer-free had the virus.

The WHO researchers found that women infected with HPV who had used birth control pills for an accumulated total of five years or more were nearly three times more likely to develop cervical cancer than HPV infected women who had never taken the pill. The increased risk persisted for up to 14 years after stopping the contraceptives. Women who had taken the pill for 10 years or more were four times more likely to get the disease than those who had never taken it. Using the pill for less than five years did not result in a higher chance of cervical cancer. The study also found that women who had taken the pill were no more likely than the others to be carriers of HPV.

That indicates that rather than enhancing the chances of getting an HPV infection or of prolonging one—as some have suspected—the pill promotes progression of the infection to cancer, said David Skegg, head of the preventive and social medicine department at the University of Otago in New Zealand who was not involved in the research.

Women have about 1 percent chance of developing cervical cancer. That means that, based on the study's findings, taking the pill for five years or more could push that chance up to about 3 percent and taking it for a total of 10 years could raise it to about 4 percent.

Worldwide, almost 360,000 women were diagnosed with cervical cancer in 1990, the latest date for which figures are available. Of those, 190,000 died of the disease. It is the second most common cancer in women. Cervical cancer strikes 12,900 American women each year and kills 4,400 of them.

(e) FDA Panel Backs Cervical Cancer Screening Test (Reuters Health—08/03/2002)

A panel of expert advisors to the US Food and Drug Administration (FDA) conditionally backed the expanded use of a human papillomavirus (HPV) DNA probe for cervical cancer screening. The FDA's Microbiology Device Panel voted 6 to 2 in favor of approving Digene Corporation's HPV DNA test Hybrid Capture 2 as a general screening test for the absence of high-grade cervical disease or cancer, when used in conjunction with a Pap smear in women aged 30 and older.

The Hybrid Capture 2 can detect 13 HPV DNA types in

cervical specimens. HPV is a common infection, affecting an estimated 75% of sexually active American adults. Often the infection goes away on its own. But infection with certain HPV strains is linked to an increased risk of cervical cancer. If the FDA should follow its committee recommendation, the test would now be indicated for helping identify women at risk for cervical cancer based upon the presence of HPV. The FDA previously cleared the first-generation hybrid DNA probe in 1995 for determining the grade of HPV-related disease in confirmed cases and to support unclear Pap smear results. The Hybrid Capture 2 is an updated version of that first-generation test.

In seeking the new indication, Digene's Chief Scientific Officer Dr. Attila Lorincz said that the company was in effect seeking to develop a new stratification system for high-risk women. At present, Lorincz noted that women are classified as either high-risk or low-risk based upon their and their partner's sexual history. Lorincz said the HPV test would provide a more objective method for identifying high-risk individuals with a negative Pap smear result. Lorincz said those women could then be followed more closely, allowing for earlier intervention. "Imagine, there are about 5,000 deaths a year due to cervical cancer. This is a highly treatable disease when caught early. There should be no deaths," Lorincz said.

Under the current American College of Obstetrics and Gynecology (ACOG) guidelines, women 30 and older are encouraged to have a Pap smear every one to three years. Women with positive results are either given a more invasive test for cervical disease or re-tested more frequently, depending upon the grade of the results.

Testifving on behalf of the company, experts said the DNA probe would also provide additional assurance to millions of women that they are at low risk for the disease. The Pap smear currently misses about 50% of patients with significant precursors for cervical cancer, observed Dr. Maureen Killackey, director of the Basset Regional Cancer Program in Cooperstown, New York. "It's clear to the public that the Pap smear is less than a perfect test," she said.

Voicing similar support for use of the test was the Association of Reproductive Health Professionals, other healthcare professionals and patient advocates. In making the recommendation, the committee had to struggle with a different interpretation of the data and its clinical implications. A total of eight studies were submitted for the panel's consideration, including six conducted outside the US and three that were conducted using an older-generation test.

The FDA said that only three of the eight tests showed a statistically significant difference in sensitivity, and due to the study differences, the data did not appear to be "poolable" across the studies to support approval of the test as a primary screening method.

Digene countered that although the absolute increase in identifying low-risk individuals varied according to the Pap results, the relative increase in sensitivity was always significant when compared to the Pap smear alone.

Panel members voting in favour of approval said they believed there was sufficient evidence to show that tests could aid detection, if coupled with the appropriate patient and physician education. "It's a good test, but we don't have the data for clinical practice," noted panel member Dr. L. Barth Reller, a professor of pathology and clinical microbiology at the Duke University Medical Center.

The panel members said the recommendations should be developed prior to approval, but that they would leave it up to the FDA to determine if additional clinical trials might be needed.

Digene CEO Evan Jones said that Digene believes new trials would not be necessary. Jones said it was the company's belief that it could work with the FDA to develop the appropriate recommendations.

The FDA often follows its committee's advice, but the agency is not bound by their votes. If the FDA approves the new indication, Lorincz said Digene expects the DNA probe to have a moderate effect on screening for cervical cancer at first with a growing influence over time. Cost of the Hybrid Capture 2 currently ranges from $ 40 to $ 70. But Lorincz said Digene anticipates that the cost would decrease due to accompanying increase in volume. ACOG, Director of Clinical Practice, Mary F. Mitchell said the organization currently is also considering incorporating the HPV test into its guidelines, but does not at this time believe that there is sufficient data to make its addition clinically relevant.

(f) Approval for New Digene Cancer Test Urged (Reuters—11/03/2002)

Irene's test for the virus that causes most cases of cervical cancer should be approved for use as a general screening test with Pap smears in women age 30 and older, a US advisory panel ruled. The gene-based test already is on the market for helping doctors and patients decide what to do when Pap smears, the standard screening tests for cervical cancer, provide inconclusive results.

Wider use of Digene's test will catch women at higher risk for cervical cancer who are missed by annual Pap smears, the company argued. Called the Hybrid Capture 2 HPV DNA Test, Digene's test looks for the human papilloma virus (HPV), a sexually transmitted virus found in about 99 percent of cervical cancers. Pap smears detect abnormal cells that may be cancerous or pre-cancerous. Members of a Food and Drug Administration (FDA) advisory committee voted 6-2 to urge agency approval for combining Digene's test with all Pap smears, not just questionable ones, in women 30 and older. Having HPV after age 30 suggests the virus may have persisted for years and is more likely to be dangerous. More than 35 million US women in that age group have Pap smears annually.

"This (test) will improve cancer detection," said Dr. George Birdsong, a pathologist at Grady Memorial Hospital and a panel member.

The test also may reassure women with normal Pap smears that they are at low risk for cervical cancer, which kills about 4,400 US women annually, Digene said. The disease is treatable if caught early but lethal in late stages.

Having HPV, however, does not always mean cancer. The infection usually clears up without causing illness, and panel members expressed concerns about how women and doctors would react to positive results. Follow-up from a positive HPV test, with a normal Pap smear, could range from conducting different tests to advising a repeat of the same tests in a year or sooner. The panel urged the FDA to require

Digene, as a condition of approval, to develop recommendations for how doctors should respond to test results and to provide educational materials for patients about what a positive HPV test means.

Digene Chairman and Chief Executive Evan Jones said the company expected it would be able to meet the panel's conditions. FDA approval for using the test with Pap smears "should help establish a new standard" for cervical cancer screening, Jones said in an interview.

Industry analysts say FDA approval for the wider use would expand significantly Digene's potential market for the product from its current indication, which covers the approximately 2 million abnormal U.S. Pap smears each year.

(g) HIV-1 Women More Susceptible to Cancer: Study (Times of India Online—14/01/2001)

According to the results of a study published in Lancet magazine, HIV-1 positive women are at increased risk of developing invasive vulvar cancer. In the USA, about 110,000-155,000 women are affected with HIV-1, and they are at an increased risk of developing pre-invasive cervical lesions, which are also known as the pre-cursor to cancer and invasive cervical cancer.

Conley and colleagues did a study in 925 women to investigate the incidence of these lesions in HIV-1 positive and HIV-1 negative women and to examine risk factors. The incidence of vulvovaginal or anal warts was 16 times higher in HIV-1 positive women than in HIV-1 negative women. Substantial information suggests an association between immunosuppression and development of warts.

Viral warts and cancer were present in 30 of 481 HIV-1 positive and four of 437 HIV-1 negative women at enrolment. 33 of 385 HIV-1 positive and two of 341 HIV-1 negative women developed vulvovaginal or perianal lesions.

At enrolment, and every 6 months thereafter, participants were interviewed and underwent gynaecological examination. This examination included visual inspection of the vulva, vagina, and perianal region, a Pap smear test, cervicovaginal lavage, cervical colposcopy, and, in some cases, biopsy.

Study participants included 319 women from HIV-AIDS clinics, 142 from methadone maintenance clinics, 282 from sexually transmitted disease clinics, and 182 from a clinic for study of heterosexual HIV transmission. Age, race and ethnic origin, income, age at first sexual intercourse, and history of cigarette smoking did not differ by much between women infected and not infected with HIV-1. However, HIV-1 positive women were significantly more likely to have had human papilloma-virus DNA detected in a lavage sample at enrolment and to have had a history of prostitution, intravenous drug use, and a sexually transmitted disease.

The incidence of vulvovaginal or perianal lesions was 16 times higher in HIV-1 positive than in HIV-1 negative women. Overall, nine of 478 HIV-1 positive women without viral warts at enrolment were subsequently diagnosed with high-grade viral warts. The number of cases of invasive carcinoma, identified in HIV-1 positive women during the study, lend support to the findings of Frisch, that malignancies associated with human papilloma virus increase in people with HIV-1.

As a result, during gynecological examination, HIV-1 positive women should have a thorough inspection of the vulva and perianal region. Women with any degree of abnormality, except for typical, visible benign lesions, should be referred for colposcopy and biopsy, so that pre-invasive or invasive disease can be ruled out.

(h) Smallpox Vaccine to Cure Cervical Cancer (Times of India Online—21/11/2001)

Scientists at the British Biotechnology firm, Xeneva Group Plc have made a major breakthrough with the discovery of a modified version of the smallpox vaccine which is being seen as an effective cure for Human Papilloma Virus (HPV). Doctors at Britain's Cancer Research Campaign are hoping that with this vaccine they will be able to curb the deadly Human Papilloma Virus from spreading in the human body and causing cervical cancer. They feel that it will boost the body's immune system against the virus enough to prevent infected cells from developing into cancerous cells.

However, the vaccine is still to be tested. Says Dr. Stephen Man, University of Wales: "We hope to recruit at least

20 women infected with the virus to see if the vaccine actually works. Each patient will be given the vaccine. Thereafter, their blood tests, and tissue samples will be examined and their immune response will be monitored to see if the vaccine is effective in any way." Dr. Man and his colleagues, Dr. Alison Fiander and Dr. Amanda Tristam are hoping that the vaccine proves to be an alternative to laser treatment and surgery, generally used to battle cancer.

HPV is a fairly common virus and nearly eighty percent of the world population of women is affected with it at some time during their lives. In most cases the immune response is sufficient enough to deal with it but in some cases, the early cells turn into cancerous cells. Although there are more than a hundred types of the Human Papilloma Virus, not every one of them causes cervical cancer. It is only types sixteen and eighteen that carry the highest risk for cervical cancer. Cervical cancer affects almost 465,000 women worldwide each year and is responsible for nearly 300,000 deaths. If diagnosed and treated in its earliest stages, this type of cancer can be cured.

Scientists are very optimistic with the discovery of this new vaccine and even before the tests are showing positive results, researchers have begun work on developing vaccines for women in advanced stages of cervical cancer. In addition to this work is on to discover preventive drugs to protect young girls from becoming infected with HPV.

(i) Common Virus may Reduce Cervical Cancer Risk (Times of India Online—08/04/2001)

A common virus may interfere with the human papillomavirus (HPV), a sexually transmitted infection linked to cervical cancer. In a new study, women with HPV who also were infected with the adeno-associated virus (AAV) were less likely to have cervical abnormalities, or lesions, that could become cancerous.

AAV may interfere with HPV to help protect women from developing pre-cancerous lesions that sometimes develop into cervical cancer. There is however a need for long-term studies to find out the precise role of AAV in women with HPV.

HPV can cause genital warts, although the infection

does not always cause symptoms. Some strains of the virus increase a woman's risk of cervical cancer. The study followed more than 300 South Carolina women, who received routine Pap smears at county health departments. Fifty-five had high-grade cervical lesions, meaning the abnormalities had a high risk of becoming cancerous; 162 women had low-grade lesions and 96 were lesion-free.

Nearly 71 per cent of women without cervical lesions and 67 per cent of women with low-grade lesions tested positive for AAV. The AAV infection was present in only about 54 per cent of women with high-grade lesions. The researchers also found that women with higher levels of AAV had a lower risk of high-grade lesions, and that high-grade lesions were most common in women who had HPV but did not have AAV.

Screening for HPV and AAV at the time of a routine Pap smear may help identify women at increased risk of developing high-grade lesions, according to the investigators. However, the relationship between AAV and HPV needs to be confirmed first. The researchers are not sure how AAV may reduce the risk of cervical lesions. More and more evidence suggests that AAV and HPV infect the same tissue in women, so the two viruses may interact in some way. AAV may interfere with high-risk HPV's ability to integrate into human cells. But the exact role of AAV remains uncertain.

If confirmed, the findings may lead to a better understanding of cervical cancer, and perhaps improved screening for and prevention of the disease. There is still no consensus on screening for HPV, which is definitely linked to cervical cancer.

(j) New Vaccine Approach may Help Treat and Prevent Pre-cancerous Lesions and Cervical Cancer (Cancer Info—28/03/2001)

A new vaccine approach may help treat and prevent pre-cancerous lesions and cervical cancer. Researchers have identified new vaccine targets for cancer-causing strains of the human papilloma virus (HPV). The scientists reported the discovery of four epitopes (protein fragments) from the virus that can induce a cellular immune response in human cells *in vitro* and may lead to an effective vaccine for treatment and prevention of cervical intraepithelial neoplasia (CIN), pre-cancerous lesions that develop into cervical cancer.

An estimated 20 million Americans are infected with HPV, a virus that is well known for causing genital warts but also accounts for over 95 percent of cervical cancer cases. CIN lesions, which precede most if not all cases of cervical cancer, occur in over 50,000 women in the United States each year. Currently, CIN is detected by Pap smear and treated by surgical removal of the pre-cancerous lesions, a costly procedure that may result in reproductive complications and requires continual post-surgery monitoring for recurrence. A vaccine is being developed that is designed to bolster the immune system against HPV, potentially providing a new way to treat and prevent both CIN and cervical cancer.

Previous research has indicated that a cellular immune response led by cytotoxic T cells is capable of controlling tumor growth and destroying virus-infected cells in HPV-infected patients. The latest research shows that it may be possible to emulate this successful immune response with a vaccine that consists of epitopes from several cancer-causing strains of HPV.

There are over 70 identified types of HPV, but only a relatively few high-risk strains, including HPV-16 and HPV-18, are known to cause CIN and cervical cancer. Scientists have identified epitopes predicted to activate cytotoxic T cells (CTLs) from several proteins of most cancer causing HPV strains. The current study showed that four epitopes from HPV-18, three derived from E6 and one derived from E7, were highly immunogenic using human cells *in vitro*, meaning they induce a CTL response. Research by others has indicated that E6 and E7 proteins are "oncoproteins" that are responsible for the transformation of HPV-infected cells into CIN and cancer cells. It is believed that a vaccine based on epitopes derived from these proteins may provide strong therapeutic benefit by teaching the immune system to recognize and attack HPV-infected cells at all stages of pre-cancerous and cancerous development.

Clinical trials of an HPV epitope-based vaccine have shown the potential benefit of this approach to treat CIN. The conformation of additional HPV epitopes, such as those identified in the current study is important in creating an effective vaccine.

The present cancer program is focused on developing vaccines for breast, colon and lung cancer as well as prostate and CIN/cervical cancer using gene maps of cancer-associated proteins and infectious agents to design vaccines that induce cellular immunity.

An extensive technology platform is based on pioneering work in deciphering the genetic code which regulates T-cell activation and identifying antigen fragments known as epitomes which can activate highly targeted T-cell responses to tumors, viruses, bacteria and parasites. This new field of pharmacology opens two significant areas of pharmaceutical development: protective vaccines that activate T-cell protection against infections, such as HIV and hepatitis C, and therapeutic vaccines designed to stimulate antigen-specific T-cell responses to infections, such as HIV, hepatitis C and hepatitis B, and tumors such as breast, colon, lung and prostate.

(k) Scientists Identify New Vaccine Targets for Cancer-causing Strains of Human Papilloma Virus (Cancer Info—28/03/2001)

A new vaccine which targets cancer-causing strains of the human papilloma virus (HPV) may help treat and prevent pre-cancerous lesions and cervical cancer. Four epitopes (protein fragments) from the virus that can induce a cellular immune response in human cells *in vitro* and may lead to an effective vaccine for treatment and prevention of cervical intraepithelial neoplasia (CIN), pre-cancerous lesions that develop into cervical cancer have been identified.

An estimated 20 million Americans are infected with HPV, a virus that is well known for causing genital warts but also accounts for over 95 percent of cervical cancer cases. CIN lesions, which precede most if not all cases of cervical cancer, occur in over 50,000 women in the United States each year. Currently, CIN is detected by Pap smear and treated by surgical removal of the pre-cancerous lesions, a costly procedure that may result in reproductive complications and requires continual post-surgery monitoring for recurrence.

The new vaccine is designed to bolster the immune system against HPV, potentially providing a new way to treat and prevent both CIN and cervical cancer.

Previous research had indicated that a cellular immune response led by cytotoxic T-cells is capable of controlling tumor growth and destroying virus-infected cells in HPV-infected patients. Research shows that it may be possible to emulate this successful immune response with a vaccine that consists of epitopes from several cancer-causing strains of HPV. There are over 70 identified types of HPV, but only a relatively few high-risk strains, including HPV-16 and HPV-18, are known to cause CIN and cervical cancer.

Epitopes predicted to activate cytotoxic T-cells (CTLs) from several proteins of most cancer causing HPV strains have been identified. The study showed that four epitopes from HPV-18, three derived from E6 and one derived from E7, were highly immunogenic using human cells *in vitro,* meaning they induce a CTL response. It is believed that a vaccine based on epitopes derived from these proteins may provide strong therapeutic benefit by teaching the immune system to recognize and attack HPV-infected cells at all stages of pre-cancerous and cancerous development.

(l) Chlamydia Infection Linked to Cervical Cancer (Cancer Info—17/01/2001)

If the message to practice safe sex weren't strong enough, consider this: a new study shows the sexually transmitted disease chlamydia increases a woman's risk of developing cervical cancer.

Chlamydia trachomatis, which strikes more than 4 million people each year, has been found to increase a woman's risk of squamous cell carcinoma of the cervix 6.6 times. The study is based on blood samples of 128 women with advanced cervical cancer in Finland, Sweden and Norway.

The human papillomavirus (HPV) is a common sexually transmitted disease closely associated with cervical cancer. Until now, there has been no clear link between chlamydia and cervical cancer, although it has been linked to pelvic inflammatory disease and infertility. An estimated 12,800 women are diagnosed with cervical cancer every year in the United States and about 4,800 will die from it. This is the first study providing evidence of an association between exposure to specific serotypes of C trachomatis and cervical cancer.

Many people may not know they have a chlamydial infection because symptoms may be mild or not present. Symptoms of chlamydia may include:

- ❑ Abnormal discharge (mucus or pus) from the vagina or penis.
- ❑ Pain while urinating.
- ❑ Fever.
- ❑ Abdominal discomfort.

In the study, women were tested for 10 types of chlamydia and three were linked to cervical cancer. Serotype G was found to increase a woman's risk by 6.6 times. Serotype D increased the risk by 2.7 times and Serotype I by 3.8 times, according to the study. Those exposed to more than one serotype also showed an increased risk. The researchers controlled for HPV and smoking, which is also a risk factor for cervical cancer.

The authors say that although the link between bacterial infections and cancer is not clear, genetic damage and the body's response to cell changes "could initiate or promote cervical carcinogenesis." These data provide additional justification for expanding chlamydial infection screening, not only to protect against pelvic inflammatory disease and infertility, but also potentially to prevent cervical cancer.

The good news from the report is that cervical cancer is one of the few diseases in which the causes are becoming clearer, although more research is needed.

(m) Cervical Cancer Study in the Shanks Province of China (Times of India—06/08/2000)

The Pap test for detecting cervical cancer is among the top success stories of modern medicine. Since the test was developed in the 1940s, the mortality rate from cervical cancer in some populations has dropped by 84%. In other parts, however these effects have yet to filter to. In developing countries where medical infrastructure cannot support expensive or complicated testing, only about 5% of the women have ever had a Pap test. As a result, cervical cancer remains one of the leading causes of death.

A new screening test, which is less expensive and can be performed in areas without sophisticated resources, must be developed. Researchers have focused on the Shanxi province in China where cervical cancer rates are 20-30 times higher than in the United States and conventional Pap tests are difficult or impossible to obtain.

2100 Chinese women between the ages of 35 and 45 were screened for whom the risk of cervical dysplasia is the highest. 6 different screening tools were investigated:

- The ThinPrep Pap test.
- Two tests for detecting evidence of infection with human papilloma virus or HPV, which is related to virtually all cases of cervical cancer. A self-test taken by the women themselves and that taken by doctors.
- Non-magnified visual inspection of the cervix.
- Fluorescence spectroscopy, which uses a laser beam to differentiate normal from abnormal tissue.
- Colposcopic examinations (magnified visualization).

Biopsies were also performed to compare the accuracy against these benchmarks.

Once data has been analyzed, researchers hope to determine which tests or combinations of tests will be most effective in different parts of the world, depending on human and financial resources.

(n) The Return of the Virus (Bombay Times—05/05/00)

The human papilloma virus, which causes most of the world's cervical cancer, also appears to cause some oral cancer, mostly tumors found in the tonsils. These tumors are, however, much less deadly than other cancers of the head and neck that are caused by the usual culprits, smoking or alcohol.

(o) Cervical Cancer Education Website Launched (Reuters Health—07/01/00)

The first Internet-based cervical cancer public education campaign was launched on 6th. The goal of the campaign is to reach 5 million women this month, designated Cervical Cancer Month, via the website. The site's launch was announced during a live web cast organized by the American Medical Women's Association, America Online, and the National Cervical Cancer Public Education Campaign.

Spokespersons with the campaign noted that each year 500,000 women are diagnosed with the cancer worldwide. The purpose of the website is to educate women as to the importance of regular Pap smear screening in the early detection of cervical cancer. The site also includes information about the link between the sexually transmitted disease human papillomavirus (HPV) and cervical cancer and the tests that are now available to test for HPV. Most cases of cervical cancer are linked to HPV infection.

"Cervical cancer is preventable," Dr. Angel Houghton of Houston, Texas, and the American Women's Medical Association told reporters. "Unclear results on Pap smear can be confirmed with HPV testing," she added. "No woman need die from this disease. It is curable if caught early," Houghton asserted.

(p) Study Backs Alternative to Pap Tests (TOI—06/01/00)

A study done in South Africa indicates that a self-test using a vaginal swab may provide an alternative to the Pap test in the battle against cervical cancer. The chief author of the study said that a single Pap smear misses about 40% of cervical disease. The self-collected sample is used to detect the presence of Human Papilloma Virus (HPV), which has been linked to the incidence of cervical cancer. It was found that the sensitivity of HPV DNA testing was equivalent to that of a Pap test at detecting high-grade cervical cancer. However, the HPV DNA tests also had higher rates of false positive results than Pap smears performed in a clinic.

(q) One Stop Screening for Cervical Cancer Auccessful (Reuters Health—16/12/99) Source: Cancer 1999:86:2659-2667

In California, cervical cancer is more than twice as common among Hispanic women than non-Hispanic whites. Part of the reason for this is poor cancer education, screening, and treatment among certain high-risk groups, but a new study suggests that these factors can be significantly improved by a new approach: one-stop education and screening at a neighbourhood church.

In the December 15th issue of the journal *Cancer*, Dr. Christina Holschneider of the University of California, Los Angeles and colleagues from there and elsewhere report on a pilot program run at an inner-city church in South Los Angeles. All non-pregnant women over 18 in the congregation who had not had a Pap smear in the last year were invited to participate in the free program, offered before and after Sunday religious services for six weeks and on three Saturdays.

The program, offered in English and Spanish, began with the women completing a survey about their health history, behaviour, and knowledge. A Pap smear was then taken and processed immediately onsite by a board-certified cytopathologist. While awaiting the test results, the women were given a short education program about cervical cancer awareness and prevention. The Pap smear results were given to each woman privately, and if needed, additional testing was done.

"Once it is more broadly implemented, this novel, single-visit approach could prove to be a major breakthrough" in attempts to decrease the rate of cervical cancer in hard-to-reach communities, the study authors conclude.

References

Landis SH, Murray T, Bolden S, Wing PA. Cancer statistics, 1998. *CA Cancer J Clin*, 1998; 48:6-29.

Devesa SS, Silverman DT, Young JL, Pollack ES, Brown CC, Horm JW, et al. Cancer incidence and mortality trends among whites in the United States, 1947-84. *J Natl Cancer Inst*, 1987; 79:701-70.

Elkas J, Farias-Eisner R. Cancer of the uterine cervix. *Curr Opin Obstet Gynecol*, 1998; 10:47-50.

Parazzini F, Chatenoud L, La Vecchia C, Negri E, Franceschi S, Bolis G. Determinants of risk of invasive cervical cancer in young women. *Br J Cancer*, 1998; 77:838-41.

Daling JR, Madeleine MM, McKnight B, Carter JJ, Wipf GC, Ashley R, *et al.* The relationship of human papillomavirus-related cervical tumors to cigarette smoking, oral contraceptive use, and prior herpes simplex virus type 2 infections. *Cancer Epidemiol Biomarkers Prev*, 1996; 5:541-8.

Maiman M, Fruchter RG, Guy L, Cuthill S, Levine P, Serur E. Human immunodeficiency virus infection and invasive cervical carcinoma. *Cancer*, 1993; 71:402-6.

CDC. 1998 guidelines for treatment of sexually transmitted diseases. *MMWR Morb Mortal Wkly Rep*, 1998; 47:1-111.

Woolf SH. Screening for cervical cancer. U.S. Preventive Services Task Force. Guide to clinical preventive services: report of the U.S. Preventive Services Task Force. 2d ed. Baltimore: Williams & Wilkins, 1996: 105-17.

American College of Obstetricians and Gynaecologists. Recommendations on frequency of Pap test screening. ACOG, committee opinion No. 152. *Int J Gynaecol Obstet*, 1995; 49:210-1.

American Academy of Family Physicians Summary of Policy Recommendations for Periodic Health Examination. *AAFP Policy Action*, 1997:1-14.

Cervical Cancer. NIH Consensus Statement, 1996; 14: 1-38.

Spitzer M. Cervical screening adjuncts: recent advances. *Am J Obstet Gynaecol*, 1998, 179:544-56.

American College of Obstetricians and Gynaecologists. New Pap test screening techniques. ACOG committee opinion No. 206. Washington, D.C.: ACOG, 1998.

Cannistra SA, Niloff JM. Cancer of the uterine cervix. *N Engl J Med*, 1996; 334:1030-8.

Cox JT. AGUS Pap smears: a follow-up strategy. *OBG Management*, July 1998:74-87.

Hines JF, Ghim SJ, Jenson AB. Prospects for human papillomavirus vaccine development. *Curr Opin Obstet Gynaecol*, 1998; 10:15-9.

4

RESPIRATORY PROBLEMS DUE TO CHANGES IN THE LIFESTYLE

S.K. JINDAL*

The lungs like many other organ systems also bear the brunt of the changed lifestyle. Whether the changes involve the food or the clothing, the transport or the housing and the personal habits or the hobbies, they are bound to affect the health including the respiratory health. The respiratory system of any living organism, including man, in fact is exposed through the act of breathing to the surroundings all the time—during both the awake and the sleep periods. Any change in the surroundings therefore, is bound to affect the lungs.

Besides the atmosphere there are many other factors related to the style of living which influence the respiratory health. Some of the important factors are enumerated in this chapter.

I. TOBACCO SMOKING

In spite of the availability of an increased evidence of the risks of smoking, the consumption of tobacco has

*Professor and Head, Department of Phlmonary Medicine, PGI, Chandigarh.

markedly increased. In India, about 30 percent of adult men smoke and another 30 percent consume non-smoking forms of tobacco. The habit is catching fast even among the women. A major concern is the prevalence of habit of tobacco use among the youth who associate smoking with the "cool image" of a modern person.

Besides its effects on the heart and other systems; tobacco smoking is an important cause of chronic respiratory symptoms, disability and death. It causes chronic cough and breathlessness, precipitates and/or aggravates asthma and predisposes to frequent respiratory infections. Prolonged consumption of tobacco is associated with chronic obstructive lung disease and several forms of respiratory cancers. Tobacco smoking is the most important preventable cause of death. For the lungs it can be rightly considered as the enemy number one.

2. ATMOSPHERIC POLLUTION

The atmosphere in which we live is influenced by the changes in our way of living. The excessive vehicular emissions which pollute the atmosphere constitute one such example. There is a tremendous, rather logarithmic increase in the number of vehicles plying on the roads. This is a direct manifestation of the modem life necessitating both the luxury and the need of vehicles. There is an obvious dependence on the private vehicles as well as the public transport systems to commute to different places. Atmospheric pollution from their emissions is an unintended problem associated with the use of vehicles. Exhausts from various industrial units especially those within the vicinity of residential areas add to the air pollution caused by the vehicular exhausts.

The respiratory system bears the main brunt of the atmospheric pollution. One can willingly choose or reject a food, a drink or a luxury, but there is no choice of the air one breathes. Whatever is present in the atmosphere air is inspired into the respiratory system. All the noxious material, gases, fumes and chemical particles are inhaled along with the air.

Air pollution causes non-specific symptoms such as the repeated throat and nose cleaning, eye and throat irritation, cough, sputum production and heaviness of the chest in about

20 percent of adults living in highly polluted zones. Children may suffer from recurrent respiratory tract infections, wheezing, bronchitis and asthma. Chronic exposures may cause more serious and chronic respiratory problems and disability.

3. SICK BUILDING SYNDROME: THE MENACE OF MODERN HOUSING

The multi-storeyed housing with a number of flats crowded together, is possibly a need of the modern times but certainly a factor adverse to the human health. The inside air is generally stale due to the closed surroundings. There is a significant pollution of the indoor air resulting from various exhausts and expired air of those living inside. The indoor air pollution could in fact be even more injurious than the outdoor air pollution.

Recognition of indoor air pollution is relatively recent. It is not uncommon to experience a feeling of 'suffocation' in a closed environment. It is often ascribed to lack of oxygen but this is not true. The composition of air is remarkably constant all over the world. There is about 79 percent nitrogen and 21 percent oxygen in the air—the other gases form a very small fraction. Carbon dioxide exhaled out of the lungs may accumulate in a closed and over-crowded place. But such an increase is usually small and temporary unless the room is really airtight. Exposure to poisonous gases such as carbon mono-oxide may occur in a closed room heated through burning of coal inside. This may in fact prove to be fatal.

What is more common in a poorly ventilated home is a vague constellation of symptoms described as the "sick-building syndrome". It is characterized by a general feeling of malaise, dizziness and irritation of mucus membranes. It may also be accompanied by nausea, itching, aches and pains. Psychological problems especially headaches, mental irritation, lack of concentration and depression are common. Compounded by loneliness, it may even lead to suicidal tendencies.

Sick building syndrome is common in small houses which are generally over-furnished. Some of the important pollutants whose indoor concentrations exceed those of the outdoor, include gases such as carbon mono and dioxides, oxides of nitrogen, organic substances, spores, formaldehyde, hydrocarbons, consumer product aerosols, radon and allergens. The sources are attributed to a variety of construction material, insulations, furnishings, adhesives, cosmetics, volatilization, house dusts, fungi, molds and other indoor products.

By-products of fuel combustion are important in houses with indoor kitchens. It is not only the burning of dried dung and wood which is responsible, but also the kerosene and liquid petroleum gas. Oxides of both nitrogen and sulphur are released from their combustion.

Smoking of tobacco in the closed environment is an important source of indoor pollution. It may not be high quantitatively, but significantly hazardous for health. There are over 4000 chemical constituents in the tobacco smoke which have been identified. Most of these chemicals are harmful for human health. Exposure to the environmental tobacco smoke occurs significantly in the children and spouses of smokers. It has been shown to be associated with an increased incidence of lung cancer, chronic bronchitis, lung function impairment and higher morbidity from bronchial asthma. It is the relationship of several medical problems with environmental tobacco smoke exposure (passive-smoking) that has compelled several countries to enforce laws either to prohibit smoking in public places and offices or to create separate areas for smokers and non-smokers.

Radon and radon decay products (called radon 'daughters') have been identified to bear a significant relationship with incidence of cancers, especially the lungs. The common indoor source is the construction material and water. Its concentration may vary from place to place and that may actually determine the variations in the prevalence of cancers at different places.

Chemical compounds such as formaldehyde, acetone, ammonia toluene, benzene and others bearing a high indoor concentration may have subtle health effects such as the increased production of sputum, eye irritation, watering and neuro-psychiatric symptoms including headaches, aches and pains. Mineral synthetic and asbestos fibres emanating from insulation and fire retardant material are quite hazardous and responsible for lung fibrosis and tumours. Asbestos fibres are non-destructible and may cause the disease after several years of the initial exposure.

Micro-organisms and allergens are of special significance in causation and spread of diseases. Most of the infective illnesses may involve more persons of a family living in common indoor environment. These include viral (such as influenza, measles) and bacterial diseases such as tuberculosis. A classic example of an epidemic due to indoor pollution was the Legionnaire's disease where the causative organisms responsible for a severe pneumonic illness, first involving members attending an American Legion Conference in Philadelphia and killing a many, was traced to the air duct system.

Other indoor air problems include the allergic problems of the respiratory system, skin and eyes. Hypersensitivity pneumonias such as the air-conditioner and water-cooler lung may result from allergens present in these fittings. Similarly, mosquitoes breeding in water coolers may spread diseases such as the malaria and the dengue fever.

The spectrum of indoor air pollution is wide and its effects devastating. It not only causes an increased morbidity and mortality from diseases but threatens the quality of life. It is apt to say that the sickness of the building is transferred to the sickness of inhabitants. The architects, the builders and the inhabitants need to look into the health of the indoor air as much as into the interior design.

4. PHYSICAL INACTIVITY

There is a great increase in sedentary habits among both the youth and the children. The marked increase in television programmes, video games and computer use has resulted in indoor confinement of people who should otherwise be out in the playgrounds, parks or fields. Furthermore, there is an excessive dependence on vehicles for transportation from place to place. Even within the campuses and large buildings, people would use motorized mechanisms, escalators, conveyor belts and lifts rather than exercising their legs. Regular exercises and games are rather limited to the few in this country.

A comparative assessment of the major risk factors for non-communicable diseases made for the three mega countries, i.e. India, Bangla Dash and Indonesia is rather revealing. The magnitude of physical inactivity was the most pronounced in India. When physical inactivity was graded as per severity, only 11 percent people had vigorous or modern activity, while 89 percent were found to possess sedentary habits. On the other hand, sedentary habits in the developed countries are found in less than 10 percent individuals.

Physical inactivity is the obvious cause of the poor development of the respiratory reserve. It results in breathlessness, respiratory deconditioning and chronic respiratory debility.

5. OBESITY

Closely related to the physical inactivity is the problem of obesity. While excessive eating especially of the fatty and junk foods is directly responsible for obesity, the lack of exercise compounds the problem. These days, there is an over-dependence on fast foods. Even the regular foods served in star restaurants and hotels contain an excess of oils and sugars. Further, the consumption of an excessive amount of desserts, sweets, chocolates and creams add to the high caloric intake. Invariably, the weight increases unless the food is balanced and calories are burnt with a good amount of exercise.

Obesity results in a significant increase in the load on the cardio-respiratory system. Breathlessness is the most common symptom. Gradually, the lungs and the heart are unable to cope up with this burden and tend to fail. While gross obesity itself can lead to respiratory failure, even milder obesity would act as a contributory factor.

Obesity is also a cause of excessive snoring due to transitory occlusion of the upper respiratory tract. It may also result in short episodes of choking and cessation of breathing during sleep—the so-called obstructive sleep apnoea syndrome.

How to Void the Problem?

'Prevention is better than cure', is a simple dictum understood by even the most ill-informed individuals. Yet, prevention is the most inadequately and inefficiently adopted practice. But there is no short-cut to the preventive steps. Health is the most valuable and precious thing in one's life. It needs preservation at all costs.

Preventive steps for respiratory health are easy to count: Avoid or stop smoking; improve both indoor and outdoor atmospheric air and avoid pollution; regular exercises, balanced food and avoidance of obesity. Many of these issues are discussed elsewhere in the book. I would dwell upon two important topics—smoking control and good physical activity.

A. Tobacco Control—Problems and Strategies

Smoking is an addiction rather than a harmless 'habit'. Nicotine, the chief constituent of tobacco, has all the characteristics of an addictive substance similar to that of other addictive agents, e.g. alcohol, marijuana, opium, etc. These are: 1. Immediate pharmacologic reward (the 'kick'); 2. Rapidly increasing tolerance to this effect (provokes increasing consumption over time); 3. Definite withdrawal symptoms on leaving and thus having a strong tendency to reuse. Over the last 20-30 years, a variety of approaches have evolved for control of tobacco consumption: (i) Group of clinic-based programmes usually with an educational and/or behavioural modification approach; (ii) Individual treatment which includes psychotherapy, behavioural modification or hypnosis; (iii) Information disseminated by the mass media; (iv) Drugs which help or reduce the withdrawal symptoms; and (v) Self-help approaches.

Broadly, tobacco control has several aspects such as the socio-behavioural, economic, medical and political. On socio-behavioural front, every effort should be made to decrease the social acceptability of smoking at home, at work places or at social gatherings. This requires a concerted effort by each member of society aided by the governmental policies and laws. Happily some welcome steps have been taken up by several state governments in promulgating laws to ban smoking in the enclosed areas such as the cinemas, the public transport, educational institutions and hospitals. The government of India does not allow smoking on domestic flights. Any advertisement of tobacco is banned on the All India Radio and the Door-Darshan. More educational programmes specially focused on the target young, non-user population are required through a patient, extensive and persuasive campaign. Our mass media, voluntary agencies, women's organizations, educational and religious bodies can play an important role in this matter.

While the gains of tobacco are seen in terms of employment generated and the revenue collected, the losses are numerous in terms of costs incurred in providing health care to people and loss of productivity caused by diseases and death from tobacco-related diseases. Use of wood in tobacco curing also has implications in the form of environmental degradation. It has been estimated that the costs of providing health care, setting up diagnostic and therapeutic facilities outweigh the apparent economic benefits from tobacco industry.

Besides the above mentioned socio-economic aspects of tobacco control, it is even more important to help an individual smoker to quit smoking. Once appropriately motivated by socio-behavioural interventions, a smoker needs some extra help to get out of this addiction. Nicotine has definite withdrawal symptoms which vary from smoker to smoker. The withdrawal symptoms include bradycardia (low heart rate), irritability, anxiety, lack of concentration and mood abnormalities, increase in appetite, weight gain and insomnia (inability to sleep). A 'craving' for nicotine is the most common cause of failure of smoking cessation. Most of these symptoms would subside in about 2 week time provided the person continues to refrain from smoking. Other forms of medical aid available in smoking cessation programmes are given below:

1. Smoking Deterrents

These substances produce an unpleasant taste in mouth in conjunction with tobacco. Silver acetate is one such established substance available in a chewing gum form in the West.

2. Nicotine Substitutes

Nicotine chewing gums, intra-dermal implants and patches for application on skin are available to help relieve the withdrawal symptoms. They are probably less harmful as they are devoid of other toxic components of tobacco smoke.

3. Several other Drugs have been used to Reverse

The withdrawal symptoms but all of them have limited roles. It is well said that reducing withdrawal symptoms does not necessarily imply a successful smoking cessation. "Smoker may continue to smoke because he gets rewarding, effects from smoking and not because he experiences withdrawal symptoms after stopping."

A strong political and administrative will is required to effectively control the tobacco use. Non-smokers' rights have to be protected in the face of now established harmful effects of "passive smoking". Tobacco control programme requires involvement of politicians, administrators, scientists, agriculturists, industrialists and in fact, of each citizen of the society.

B. Exercise and Physical Activity

Both the lungs and the heart have a tremendous potential of increasing their activities in response to a stress. The volume of air breathed by the lungs and the blood pumped by the heart per minute can expand several fold during exercise. This obviously puts a great strain on the system. But the relative increase shall differ in those who are accustomed to exercise, than those who are not. Therefore, the symptoms of stress are tolerated much latter by the acclimatized people. Athletes, sportsmen and those who exercise regularly have slower heart and respiratory rates. Their lung capacities are higher and blood pressures towards the lower limits of the normal. They have therefore, a much greater scope of improving their functions in case of an unaccustomed event.

Exercise not only helps in avoiding symptoms but keeps the mood elevated. It helps in building confidence and removing mental fatigue and tension. It is of special importance for students when their studies are hard and time-consuming. A short period of play goes a long way in improving literary performance.

Physical exercise is also essential for normal activities of neuromuscular system, joints and bones. It helps to increase the blood circulation and develop collateral supplies to different organs. This not only helps in prevention of diseases such as heart attack and osteoporosis, but also promotes better control of diseases such as asthma, diabetes and hypertension. It is important here to warn that exercise in the presence of a disease must be undertaken only under guidance of the treating physician. Any exercise is an additional burden, which, a diseased organ may not be able to cope with. It may be counter-productive in diseases of the lungs, heart and the joints. For example, it is a common misnomer among people that respiratory exercises are good for all lung diseases. This is not true. Exercise consumes excess oxygen, which a diseased lung may not be able to contribute.

Therefore, exercise for patients with medico-surgical diseases, need to be regulated. In some, it is required to be restricted forever, in others, a clearly structured programme is essential for rehabilitation. Exercise-prescription in patients has to be specific for its type, intensity, duration and frequency. Further, the progression from mild to moderate and severe exercises need to be gradual and guided by the body's response. There is no reason as to why a patient should not resume normal lifestyle and physical activities. This is essential for a good quality of life. But this cannot be allowed at the cost of disease control. Obviously, most patients are keen to go back to a state of normal physical activity. But this may or may not be achieved. It also depends on the disease state, the patient's enthusiasm and understanding. Above all, it is the patient's pre-morbid level of exercise which determines the outcome. A person who had been less active, physically in health before, would continue to remain shy after the illness. The fact of the matter is that exercise is far more important in health than in disease.

The patients of cancer cervix on chemotherapy treatment say they are "bone-tired". Simple things like taking a bath or even eating a full meal are exhausting. Most cancer patients will feel this extreme fatigue for weeks or months. This feeling is considered the No. 1 side effect of cancer and largely is caused by the chemotherapy or radiation necessary to fight the disease. Yet few patients seek or receive treatment for fatigue. Studies suggest that over 75 percent of cancer patients suffer serious fatigue. It limits their ability to work, attend school or perform daily activities. There is a mental toll where patients cannot concentrate, are forgetful or depressed. It even can hinder rigorous cancer therapy. Part of the problem is dispelling the myths that there is no help for fatigue, or that fatigue only could mean the cancer is worsening so patients are scared to mention it. Anemia is a leading culprit, because radiation and many powerful chemotherapy drugs that kill cancer cells also kill blood and bone marrow cells. Medicines, such as Epogen or Procrit, that boost blood-cell production or blood transfusions may help. Under treated pain is another big cause, limiting patients sleep. Some new studies suggest mild exercise programs help, because constant rest actually makes patients quickly lose muscle strength, thus worsening fatigue. Tumors can compete for a body's nutrients at the same time that chemotherapy-caused nausea depletes calories and spurs dehydration. There are medicines to minimize nausea, and nutritionists may suggest easier-to-tolerate, high-nutrient meals. Sometimes help can be creative. Put a chair under the shower or a roiling stool in the kitchen to conserve energy. The attending doctor may not fully understand the degree of fatigue and that is frustrating to patients, as is finishing treatment and still being fatigued.

5

SMOKING: AVOIDABLE CHALLENGE TO YOUR FITNESS AND HEALTH

To put it simply, smoking has struck the human race like a disaster; only difference is that it doesn't exhibit its devastation suddenly. Fortunately, it gives enough time to put your pernicious lifestyle in back gear; you can kick the habit whenever you decide to do so and get back to the road of healthy and stress-free living. How and why, the consumption of tobacco, a patently toxic and hazardous substance started is not well known, but story goes that Portuguese sailors brought it to India in 16th century and offered it to the then Emperor 'Akbar the Great'. The emperor and his advisers didn't understand the potential risks and hazards to health and accepted the gift—thus started the wildfire in India. It started as a *hookah*, but then many other forms of inhaling the smoke of this potential carcinogen started and then several other lethal intoxicants gained ground for inhalation, what is now called substance-abuse or drug-abuse.

1. TOBACCO HAS COME TO STAY: IT CAN'T BE WISHED AWAY

Now tobacco is being used either as an inhalant or a food by 45% of Indian men and 12% of Indian women, the number of youngsters is not exactly known. Smoking cigarettes or consumption of tobacco in other ways has now become an individual, social and routine menace and is no more a ceremonial or formal occurrence.

1.1 Tobacco is Full of Poisons

Tobacco contains thousands of chemicals, out of which 600 substances can cause cancer. Three main poisons are:

(i) Tar

A solid irritant that coats the teeth, lungs and blocks the airway.

(ii) Nicotine

An addictive substance. Each cigarette contains 1mg of nicotine, known to cause heart disease.

(iii) Carbon Monoxide

It gets bound to the blood, denying it oxygen, can cause heart and vessel diseases.

Other significant poisons are formaldehyde, ammonia and benzene. It is the chief cause of avoidable, premature deaths and ill-health. 30 lakhs of smokers die each year, many more are taken ill. Lung cancer and heart disease are the main causes of death. It also causes cancer of mouth, esophagus, larynx, bladder, and pancreas, brain-stroke, chronic bronchitis, etc. Respiratory troubles, stomach upsets, Gum problems are commonly responsible for ill-health. It is also responsible for complications of pregnancy, impotence, premature ageing and reduced fertility. In heart disease, nicotine and carbon-monoxide both contribute substantially.

1.2 Why Smoking gets started and then continues?

Children start smoking due to:

(i) Peer pressure,
(ii) Desire to rebel, and
(iii) Curiosity, despite the unpleasant feelings it evokes.

Most smokers misbelieve that despite smoking health and psychic problems will not come to them (only others will suffer) and that it can be stopped anytime, much before problems could start. It does not happen in real life. Why people continue to smoke, despite the awareness of ill-effects, the reasons could be: drug dependence, enjoyment, relaxation, concentration, weight control, mood control, and fear of failure. Most of these patients have misbelieves and myths and not reasons real enough to believe.

However, on stopping smoking, reversal of process starts and if no permanent damage has occurred, one can regain lost health. 'Determination' is the keyword. Nicotine replacement therapy may be tried as skin patch, chewing gum, nasal spray, etc. If you can't stop it altogether start the process of systematic withdrawal. Exercise and diet program may help. Sometimes hypnosis and acupuncture may also work.

1.3 You can also suffer due to others' faults: Passive Smoking

Passive smoking is the inhaling of smoke by non-smokers from the smoke filled atmosphere. Non-smokers inhale the side stream smoke that is not drawn through the cigarette. Their lungs filter smoke, which is exhaled by the smokers. But the undiluted side stream smoke contains much higher percentage of tar, nicotine and noxious gases than inhaled smoke. The non-smokers are frequently exposed to such second-hand smoke at home, during travel or in the workplace. It may cause breathing difficulties in some and trigger allergic reactions in others. It is also dangerous for people with certain kinds of heart diseases. Increased risk of lung cancers is found in the non-smoking wives of cigarette smokers. Due to second-hand smoke, the children of the smokers may develop asthma, allergic rhinitis, etc. They also become more prone to respiratory tract infections and ear infections. It may also result in sudden infant death syndrome. Smoking in pregnant woman may lead to low birth weight baby, still-births, and fatal malformations.

1.4 Various Deadly Forms of Tobacco—Avoid Them All

Tobacco can be smoking variety or smokeless variety. It can be inhaled, chewed or swallowed, in different forms. Tobacco smoking is a widespread habit in most cultures and societies throughout the world. Tobacco is smoked either as a cigarette, cigar or in a pipe. Modified cigarette brands are used in local areas. These include:

(a) Indian Bidi

It consists of shredded, sun-dried tobacco in small quantity that is hand-rolled into a piece of tendu. These are popular in India. It is seen that bidi smoking starts at an early age among the school children and locals. It is associated with high rate of oral pre-cancerous lesions among the users. The local brands differ from regions to regions. In India, different forms of chewing tobacco are used such as khaini, pattiwala tobacco, maiwpuri tobacco, zarda, kiwam and gadakhu.

(b) Khaini

This is powered tobacco mixed with slake lime paste, sometimes used with areca nut. It is placed inside the mouth. Indonesian Kretek is characterized by the addition of cloves, which gives an aromatic quality to the cigarette smoke. In Indonesia, tobacco may be wrapped in the corn or in banana leaves. *New Guinea's stick* consists of locally grown tobacco that is shredded and rolled in coarse paper such as newspaper or in a modern cigarette paper. The commercially manufactured cigarettes are made of fine cut tobacco wrapped in a paper. This tobacco is generally treated with sugars, flavoring agents and aromatic substances. Cigars are of various sizes and comprise of both imported and made in India.

(c) Chuta

This is a home-made cigar in Andhra Pradesh where it is a popular habit and may begin in childhood. It is made of tobacco wrapped in dried tobacco leaf. In some areas of the state it is smoked with the lighted end in the mouth. This is described as reverse smoking. Cigarillo consists of cigar tobacco wrapped in treated cigarette paper. It is also called as cigarette like cigar. Churat is a small cigar made of heavy-bodied cigar tobacco. Khiyo Cigars are the locally produced cigars in Thailand. Commercially manufactured cigars consist of cigar tobacco wrapped in a tobacco leaf paper or the reconstituted tobacco.

(d) Pipe-smoking

Pipe smoking was one of the earliest forms of tobacco smoking. Local variations of pipe smoking are found throughout the world. In India chillum is used, while in Nepal sulpa is used. Water pipe, which has also known as hookah, goza or sheesha is used in Middle-East, Asia (Rural India) and parts of Africa. Piped tobacco found locally is of variable composition. The commercially manufactured forms of pipe tobacco consist of blended tobacco to which sugar and flavouring agents are added. People who smoke cigars or pipes suffer fewer harms from smoke inhalation than those who smoke cigarettes do.

(e) Pattiwala Tobacco

It is a sun-cured tobacco leaf. It may be used with or without lime. On the other hand, Maiwpuri tobacco consists of a mixture of tobacco, slacked lime, areca nut and spices. Mishri is powdered tobacco which is dark roasted.

(f) Zarda

This is used in India and Arab countries. Tobacco leaf is boiled with spices and lime till evaporation. Residual tobacco is then dried and coloured and then consumed. Kiwami is destalked tobacco leaf, which is boiled in rose water to which spices are added. It is then used as thick paste. It can be further dried and used as granules or pills.

Gudakhu includes a paste of powdered tobacco molasses and other ingredients. Other forms of chewing tobacco used in different countries are Shammah, nass, and naswar. Shammah is used in Saudi Arabia. It is a mixture of powdered tobacco leaf, lime carbonate and other ingredients. Nass is used in Iran and Central Asia. It consists of mixture of tobacco, cotton ash or sesame oil, lime and gum. Naswar is the form of chewing tobacco that is widely used in Afghanistan, Pakistan and India. It is a mixture of powdered tobacco, slacked lime and indigo. Some of the forms such as khaini, mishri, nass, naswar, shammah are just placed in the mouth and not chewed. While other forms such as zarda are chewed. Mishri and gutaka are used as tooth cleaning agents. The non-chewed tobacco is mostly kept along the gum behind the lip.

(g) Snuff

This form of Naswar is used as inhalant in India. Snuff is finely powdered plant material. The plant principally used is tobacco. Snuff is either used plain or mixed with other agents. It may be used orally or nasally.

The composition and usage varies in every region. In North America snuff is just placed in the mouth along the gum in the lip fold or the buccal fold. Sometimes it is placed under the tongue. In India, it is used as tooth-cleaning agent also. A moist type of snuff is available in North America and Europe. It consists of finally cut tobacco, which is pulverized and used either orally or nasally. In South Africa oriental snuff is used. This consists of tobacco, gum, white earth and water. The snuff is produced by sun-drying this mixture.

(h) Gutka, the Smokeless Tobacco

In India, an emerging trend in tobacco consumption is the development of new smokeless tobacco products such as gutka which is widely consumed by women and children. Gutka is a sweetened mixture of tobacco, betel and catechu, which is chewed together. It is then spat out. It is sold in small brightly coloured packets that attract children. Chewing tobacco is more likely to cause mouth cancer. This is because the tobacco is in the concentrated form and held in the mouth for a longer period of time. More and more children are consuming gutka as the small coloured sachets easily attract them. These sachets are cheaper than sweets and easily available. Some children as young as 12 years, show pre-cancerous lesions of the mouth after regular use of gutka.

Education and awareness among the population in general and youth in particular about the injurious effects of tobacco on health is the most important measure. The users should be made aware of the ill-effects of tobacco use and that it kills in the long-run. Every smoker should give up smoking even if he/she has been smoking for a long time as cessation prevents further damage to the health. Worth trying are other things such as carrot sticks, hiding ash-trays, long walks, making friends, developing athletic skills, weight control, spending time in places where smoking is not permitted such as a library. In India, there is a ban on smoking at all public places, but it is being violated with impurity.

2. SMOKING ATTACKS YOUR FITNESS

It is a well-known fact that smoking attacks your fitness in a number of ways and at almost all the organs, chiefly by reducing the amount of oxygen available in the body. Since oxygen plays a major role in energy production, even a minor depletion has an impact on physical and mental well-being and performance of entire human system. The major effects of smoking on the body's respiratory and circulatory systems are: (i) Caron monoxide from smoking reduces the amount of oxygen absorbed from the lungs, (ii) Carbon monoxide in the blood also reduces the amount of oxygen released from the blood for various organs and systems, (iii) Smoke inhalation has an immediate effect on respiration, increasing airways resistance. Smoking causes chronic (or long-term) swelling of mucous membranes, which also leads to increased airways resistance, and (iv) Smoking increases the heart rate for a given level of exercise and reduces its efficiency.

2.1 The Main Offender

Carbon monoxide (the same lethal gas which is released by motor vehicle exhausts) is present in cigarette smoke and is absorbed rapidly into the bloodstream. Though oxygen has a great affinity for haemoglobin, carbon monoxide has a much greater affinity (200 to 300 times greater than oxygen) and so binds preferentially to haemoglobin. Therefore, as the level of carbon monoxide in the blood increases, the level of oxygen decreases. This has a significant effect on heart and other muscle cells where there is a high demand for oxygen. Blood levels of carbon monoxide from smoking can also produce distortions of time perception, psychomotor and visual impairment, negative effects on cognitive skill and sports performance.

2.2 Effects on the Lungs

Inhaling cigarette smoke results in airways resistance (narrowing of air passages) in the bronchi and lungs within seconds. Smoking also causes chronic swelling of the mucous membranes of the airways, which adds to airways resistance and consequent less oxygen to blood in the circulation. The tar in cigarette smoke adds to airways resistance. This tar coats the lungs, reducing the elasticity of the air sacs and resulting in the absorption of further less oxygen into the bloodstream. Tar also affects the cleansing mechanism of the lungs, allowing pollutants to remain in lungs. Increased phlegm and coughing, and damage to the cilia (the hair-like projections which "sweep" pollutants out of the airways) are the result.

2.3 Effects on the Heart

The combined effect of carbon monoxide and increased airways resistance causes the heart to work harder in an attempt to compensate for the lack of oxygen reaching the muscles. The nicotine in cigarette smoke also acts as a stimulant, increasing the heart rate and blood pressure, and decreasing the flow of blood through the blood vessels. This reduced availability of blood and oxygen to different muscle groups, reduces physical endurance and impedes physical performance. It also increases fatigue during and after exercise. In a study it was found that adolescents who had smoked for five days had an 8% reduction in endurance time compared to controls.

2.4 Attitudes to Fitness—Australian Studies

There have been several Australian studies which have assessed the attitudes among smokers. Unfortunately, many persons engaged in exercises and fitness activities also smoke, thus reducing their fitness levels. Many students agree that smoking affects their sporting ability, but still they continue smoking. Those who give up smoking, find improvements. In a study, 40% of males and 28% of females saw improved fitness as an important advantage. In another study, smokers were found to be more likely to drink alcohol and not participate in regular exercise than non-smokers or ex-smokers.

2.5 Save your Kids from Tobacco

Tobacco use usually begins in early adolescence, typically by age 16. Almost all first use occurs before young people leave high school. If adolescents can be kept tobacco-free, most will remain tobacco-free for the rest of their lives. Smoking is common among 17-18 years old (more than 25% of these young people smoke and drink and many take to harder drugs and unprotected sex). Adolescent tobacco use is also associated with being in quarrels, fights, carrying and use of weapons.

The younger a person begins smoking, the greater the risk for developing the numerous problems and illnesses associated with smoking viz., decrease in physical fitness, increased coughing and phlegm, susceptibility and severity of respiratory illnesses, development of artery disease (a possible precursor of heart disease) slower rate of lung growth—and by adulthood possible reduced level of normal lung function. Nicotine addiction makes quitting smoking as hard as quitting heroin, cocaine or alcohol. For most smokers, nicotine addiction begins during childhood or adolescence. Earlier it begins, more harmful effects, it causes in a cumulative manner, also more difficult to leave the habit.

2.6 Smokeless Tobacco

Smokeless tobacco is definitely not safe. Smokeless tobacco is as dangerous as the cigarettes. Adolescent users of smokeless tobacco have early signs of gum disease, develop lesions in their oral soft tissue (a possible warning sign of cancer), may become cigarette smokers again. Advertisements in print media, T.V. banners, etc. all influence the young minds. All publicity and all glamourisation of tobacco use should be stopped by the State and the Society joined together.

2.7 Nicotine is the Culprit—An Addiction Indeed!

Nicotine is one of the most addictive substances on earth, and most people who try to quit cigarettes will have a hard time. The chemical goes directly from the lungs to the brain and stimulates the production of dopamine, a chemical that makes you feel happy. Although nicotine can make you feel more energetic when you start smoking, your body will need more and more of it to feel the same way. If you quit, you find the craving to light up almost unbearable, and you're likely to get headaches and feel tired, sleepy, hungry, or irritable. In fact, many people attempt to quit smoking every year, but only 7 percent of them succeed. Follow the examples of successfully quitters.

Some people believe smoking lifts the spirits, but in reality it can sink your mood. If you're already down or depressed, cigarettes can put you at higher risk for clinical depression, hyperactivity, and attention deficit disorder, according to a recent report. Teens who smoke are four times as likely to be depressed as teens who don't. Smoking isn't safe even if you're smoking one cigarette a day. Every cigarette contains about 1 to 2 milligrams of nicotine, and it reaches your brain 10 seconds after you inhale. Immediately after that first puff, you'll get a rush of adrenaline that may increase your blood pressure, your heart rate, and your breathing.

Smoking causes a number of other lung diseases, including emphysema, a degenerative disease that makes breathing more and more difficult. Smoking also increases your risk of heart disease, particularly if you have high blood pressure or high cholesterol, and aggravates many digestive disorders as well. It can also cause causer of the mouth, larynx (voice box), and esophagus. Smoking also plays a role in cancer of the pancreas, kidney, bladder, and, in women, cancer of the cervix. There is no truth in the statement that smoking lowers your blood pressure and brings relaxation of mind

2.8 You can Stop Smoking—Many others have done it

Smoking stains your teeth, causes wrinkles on your face, and puts cigarette burns in your clothes. It won't do wonders for your breath or your body aroma, either. In a recent poll, most girls said they'd rather date a non-smoker than a smoker. Moreover, studies show that men with high blood pressure who smoke are far more likely than non-smokers to become impotent. That's not exactly sexy. It's true that many smokers gain weight once they stop smoking. Many of them substitute eating for the oral gratification that comes from puffing on a cigarette. On average, quitters gain only 5 to 10 pounds. But once you've stopped smoking, the weight gain doesn't have to be permanent. In fact, if you exercise, you may not only lose the weight you've gained, you may increase the stamina and lung capacity you lost when you were smoking. To help you keep the weight-off, replace smoking with other activities (instead of eating): chewing gum, doodling, sucking on a straw, or just stretching and breathing deeply. Stop smoking can enhance your life and add quality to it.

3. HEART DISEASE IS THE COMMONEST CAUSE OF DEATH AMONG SMOKERS

Most people think that lung cancer is the disease most commonly associated with smoking. However, it is actually diseases of the heart and cardiovascular system which are the major causes of death for smokers. Smoking is believed to be the most important preventable risk factor for coronary heart disease (CHD) in India. Of a large number of deaths due to smoking in India each year, more than 36% are from smoking-attributable heart attacks. This association is even stronger in younger adults, with smoking implicated in as many as 75% deaths from heart attack in this group.

3.1 How Smoking Affects the Heart?

Of thousands of chemical substances identified in cigarette smoke, the most damaging to the cardiovascular system are nicotine and carbon monoxide (immediate and long-term effects). Nicotine results in immediate and transient increases in blood pressure, heart rate, cardiac output and coronary blood flow, and causes narrowing of arteries in the legs. These effects can be fatal if narrowing of blood vessels and hardening of artery walls is already present. Carbon monoxide binds to haemoglobin, thus reducing the amount of oxygen delivered to the tissues. There is a cumulative effect of these assaults. Smoking may repeatedly damage the lining of blood vessels and encourage clot formation. This contributes to the development of atherosclerosis which can lead to raised blood pressure and increased clot formation.

3.2. Heart Attacks—Several other Problems

Coronary heart disease (CHD) is the top killer. The

death rate for smokers is about 70% higher than for non-smokers. For very heavy smokers, the risk is 200% higher. Smokers run three times the risk of sudden death compared with non-smokers. One of the causes of sudden death is ventricular fibrillation which prevents the heart beating effectively.

Aortic aneurysm is a ballooning of the aortic artery wall at the point of the artery weakened by the pressure from blood flow. This aneurysm can rupture, with life-threatening consequences. For smokers, the risk of a ruptured aortic aneurysm is upto eight times that for non-smokers. Stroke or cerebrovascular accident, is an interruption of blood supply to the brain, which can result from atherosclerosis or high blood pressure. Smoking is a contributing factor, especially in younger people. Peripheral vascular disease is a disease of the blood vessels in the legs caused by atherosclerosis. Cigarette smoking is the most important risk factor for this disease, which is rarely found in non-smokers. Peripheral vascular disease can lead to painful leg ulcers which are slow to heal and eventually lead to gangrene, resulting in amputation of the limb.

High blood pressure (hypertension) combined with smoking greatly increases the risk of coronary heart disease. Malignant hypertension is more common in smokers than non-smokers. Women who take the contraceptive pill and also smoke, face up to 39 times greater risk of having either a heart attack or stroke than women who neither smoke nor take the pill.

A 30% increase in the risk of heart attack for the non-smoker spouses of smokers, has been found in a study, revealing the perils of passive smoking. A smoker's risk of coronary heart disease and other ailments increase with the number of cigarettes smoked each day, the total number of years the smoker has smoked and the degree to which smoke is inhaled.

Smoking cessation is beneficial, even after cardiovascular disease has developed. Smokers who stop smoking after they survive their first heart attack greatly reduce their risk of dying subsequently from cardiovascular disease.

4. BRAIN STROKE—A SCENARIO OF LOSS OF SPEECH AND PARALYSIS OF LIMBS

Smokers are more likely to develop a cerebral thrombosis [stroke] than non-smokers. Sub-arachnoid haemorrhage [a form of stroke] is more common in smokers, especially women who also take the contraceptive pill. Female smokers who use contraceptive pills are many times more likely to suffer a stroke than female non-smokers who do not use contraceptive pills.

5. PERIPHERAL VASCULAR DISEASE (PVD)—VESSELS IN THE LIMBS ALLOW LESS BLOOD

There are thousands of limbs amputated each year due to peripheral vascular disease caused by smoking. More than 90% of people who suffer from intermittent claudication—the pain associated with atherosclerosis or PVD in the legs—have smoked at least 20 cigarettes a day for 20 years or more. Very few are lifelong non-smokers. Buerger's Disease is a rare form of PVD, which is virtually always due to heavy smoking. Few sufferers are able to stop smoking and many of them have multiple operations, leading to the amputation of both legs. Smokers who suffer peripheral vascular disease and continue to smoke are more likely to develop gangrene than smokers who quit smoking after being diagnosed as having peripheral vascular disease. Many of them die in young age.

6. ANEURYSM—VESSEL WALL GIVES WAY

A weakness in the wall of an artery leads to a balloon-like swelling called an aneurysm. Aneurysms may eventually cause the affected artery to burst or clot, resulting in death or severe illness. Smokers are up to eight times more likely to die from a ruptured aneurysm of the abdominal aorta than non-smokers. Young teenage boys and girls who don't know the health risks of smoking or see their parents, teachers, matinee idols, friends are more likely to become regular smokers than those who are aware of the health risks. Children who smoke suffer more respiratory problems than children who do not smoke. Children in families where there are smokers suffer more coughs and respiratory infections than the children (in families) where there are no smokers.

7. CANCER AND SMOKING GO HAND IN HAND

We have mentioned elsewhere that smoking and chewing of tobacco is responsible for a large number of cases of cancers viz., lung, mouth, tongue, stomach, intestine, cervix, kidney, etc. Thus, it is known beyond doubt that tobacco contains carcinogens and can trigger cancer in any part of the body, especially where the concentration of the chemicals and pollutants is high.

7.1 What causes Cancer?

The cause of many cancers are not yet known. Cancer cannot be caught. It is not infectious like a cold or the flu. Most cancers seem to be caused by our lifestyle habits and recreation or by substances in our environment that affect our bodies, e.g. use of tobacco in any form, especially smoking. Major causes of cancer are thought to include smoking, sun exposure and UV rays, poor diet, chemicals and asbestos.

7.2 What body parts Cancer affect?

Cancer can affect all body parts except the hair, nails and teeth. Cancer is more common in some parts of the body than others, e.g. skin, lung, bowel, cervix of uterus and breast. The blood can also be affected by cancer. Cancer of the blood is called leukaemia.

7.3 How can I reduce my chances of getting Cancer?

- avoiding unnecessary exposure to the sun,
- being a non-smoker and avoiding breathing the smoke from another's cigarette (passive smoking),
- eating plenty of fresh seasonal fruit and vegetables,
- cutting down on fatty, greasy foods,
- avoiding exposure to chemicals, pollution and radiation,
- regular exercises, and

- managing your stress properly.

7.4 How is Cancer Treated?

(i) Surgery—the cancerous tissue may be cut out by a surgeon.
(ii) Radiotherapy—a beam of high-energy radiation destroys the cancer cells and can affect some normal cells as well, producing some side effects.
(iii) Chemotherapy—chemicals are used to destroy cancer cells. This treatment may also have side effects and affect other parts of the body.
(iv) Combination therapy—this may involve all, some or a combination of some of the above processes.
(v) If cancer is detected and treated at an early stage there is a greater chance of a cure and possibly less extensive treatment.
(vi) Doctors who specialize in the area of cancer and called oncologists.

8. LUNG CANCER: A WARRANT OF DEATH FOR THE SMOKER

Lung Cancer is one of the most common form of malignancy in males and rapidly increasing in females, in India. Although, the incidence is lower as compared to Western figures, in view of our larger population size the overall burden is enormous. This increase is mostly reflective of a true increase because of increased smoking in this country. Other factors like increased awareness and availability of good diagnostic facilities might be other responsible causes of the recognition of this entity. A lot of advancement has taken place in the field of the biology of lung cancer particularly the genetic aspects of lung cancer. The situation is worse in developing countries including India. Usually there is a negative attitude towards this disease from the very beginning. In view of the costly and toxic drugs used for the treatment of this disease, most of our patients do not opt for chemotherapy, which is the only available form of treatment as most of them present in advanced stage. The Government of

India and the Hon'ble Supreme Court of India have taken significant steps towards banning of smoking in public places. However, it is a long way to go to stop smoking in this country.

8.1 Indian Scenario

In India Lung cancer was initially thought to be extremely infrequent. Lung cancer constituted 14.4% of all cancers in a review of 9210 autopsies by Banker in 1957. The National Cancer Registry Programme of the Indian Council of Medical Research, which collected data from six different parts of the country, both rural and urban areas, showed varying figures at different areas. While cancer of the trachea, bronchus and lungs was the most common form of malignancy in males in 1989 from Bombay, Delhi and Bhopal. It was the second most common in Madras and third in Bangalore, and was most unusual in Barshi, a rural area. The disease was most uncommon in females and only in Bombay it was the sixth common malignancy. 40% of patients of lung cancer are less than 50 years of age and 11% are less than 40 years. In younger age group lung cancer is commonly misdiagnosed as tuberculosis.

While describing the largest series of clinical spectrum of primary lung cancer in India from Chandigarh, Jindal and Behera (1990) reported that both the mean and peak ages of lung cancer were lower compared to the West (54.3 years). The smoker to non-smoker ratio was 2.7:1. Most of the patients had advanced disease and 51.8% had evidence of metastases. The commonest presentation was mass lesion with or without collapse in 68%, 25% had pleural effusion and 16.7% had superior vena caval compression syndrome. Squamous cell carcinoma is found in 34.3%, anaplastic in 27.6%, adenocarcinoma in 25.9% and unclassified in 12.2%.

There is a wide variation in different signs and symptoms. Most of the symptoms of lung cancer mimic pulmonary tuberculosis. However, some symptoms like chest pain, mediastinal symptoms like dysphagia, hoarseness and SVC syndrome are common for lung cancer, but rare for tuberculosis. Further, clubbing, haemorrhagic pleural effusion, collapse or mass lesion on clinical examination will help the physician to think about malignancy rather than tuberculosis.

8.2 What causes Lung Cancer?

The single most major cause of lung cancer is smoking, which we have discussed earlier. The association has been well established. Tobacco has been associated with cancer for at least 200 years and the nature of the association with lung cancer has been reported for decades. Tobacco smoking is at present the most clearly defined and important cause of cancer in developed countries with lung cancer being the leading tobacco-related cancer. More than 80 percent of the cases of lung cancer are due to smoking only. Cigarettes smoking also enhances the carcinogenic effect in certain occupations, like asbestos workers, and uranium miners, compared to that in non-smokers with the same occupation. The risk is almost 14 times for the former and 5 times more in the later. Quiting smoking reduces the risk of lung cancer regardless of duration of smoking or the quantity smoked per day. It decreases slowly over 10-20 years, and after 20 years, the risk is the same to that in a non-smoker. Besides, cigarettes, cigars, and pipes, bidi, smoking is an important cause of lung cancer.

As mentioned above, damage to the lungs accumulates with continuous smoking, and therefore duration of smoking is directly related to the development of lung cancer. In fact, to express this relationship a smoking index is described. Smoking index is expressed as the number of bidis or cigarettes smoked per day multiplied by the number of years smoked. It is graded as mild, when the smoking index is below 100; moderate when it is between 100 to 299; and severe when it is 300 or more. As the smoking index increases the risk of lung cancer is also increased.

8.3 Occupational Hazards

Occupational respiratory carcinogens are several. Asbestos is by far the most important, and may account for as many as 5% of deaths from lung cancer. Apart from mining the hazards are all more prevalent in industrial towns. Studies suggest an association between exposure to silica and an excess of pulmonary malignancies. Clinical evidences suggest a link between exposure to radiation and lung cancer. The agents responsible are radon and uranium. The combining effect of gamma radiation and smoking appears to be additive. Occupational exposures have been estimated to account for 5-36% of the lung cancers among men in different areas in the West.

Occupational Risk of Lung Cancer

Agent	*Occupation*	*Comment*
1. Definitely known		
Asbestos	Shipyard Workers	Some increase in risk after 10 years. Substantial after 20 years. Smoking increases risk 90 folds.
Arsenic	Smelter workers Vineyard workers	More in upper lobes. Dose related. May have multiple primaries.
Nickel	Refinery workers	Squamous cell type common.
Radiation	Uranium mining Haematite mining, Hard rock mining	Majority oat cell type. Due to radon exposure
Chromium	Chromium ore processing Pigment manufactures	Mostly squamous cell type
Chloromethyl ethers	Workers in industries producing these compounds.	Oat cell common
Mustard gas	Mustard gas producing workers	Squamous and undifferentiated cell carcinomas more common.
Soots, tars, oils, coke	Coke oven workers Gas house workers, roofers rubber workers	

8.4 Food may Contribute

There is increasing evidence that some dietary factors may be protective for lung cancer, and some may increase the risk. Although most consistent evidence relates to a protective effect of β-carotene, some more recent work suggests that other protective factors may be found in vegetables. The risk for developing cancer is significantly increased when smoking is combined with a deficiency of vitamin. A recent case control study of diet and lung cancer in South India has shown that green vegetables and bananas have a protective association with lung cancer. Pumpkins and onions have the most consistent protective effect. Animal protein foods and diary products have a predisposing effect on lung cancer. Dietary chloesterol and animal fat increase the risk of lung cancer.

8.5 Pollution of Environment

Urban air contains several known lung carcinogens including asbestos and arsenic, and hydrocarbons from incomplete combustion of fuel. The nature of these pollutants varies and fluctuates over time, and the concentration may be affected by a number of known and unknown factors like ventilation and human responses, etc.

8.6 Chronic Lung Diseases

Individuals with chronic non-neoplastic lung diseases have a documented high risk to develop lung cancer, e.g. tuberculosis, pneumonia, emphysema. It is reported that lung cancer in association with chronic lung diseases results due to an impaired lung ventilation and concomitant increase in pulmonary carbon dioxide, which in turn may contribute to the increased burden of lung cancer in individuals with chronic lung diseases.

8.7 Predisposition

Since vast majority of heavy smokers do not develop lung cancer, it seems that an inherited predisposition exists. Although smoking is the major cause of lung cancer, only about 10 percent of heavy smokers die of this disease. The relative susceptibility of these 10% or the resistance of the remaining 90% to development of lung cancer is poorly understood and may be relative to genetic events.

9. HOW TO STOP SMOKING?

According to the ICMR report, India is the 4th largest producer of tobacco. It ranks second in the world after China in cigarette and bidi production. There are 18.4 crore users in India with 4 crore cigs., 8 crore bidis and 6 crore using chewable forms of tobacco. 45% of Indian men and 12% of women use some form of tobacco. Tobacco kills 90 persons per hour, 2200 per month and 800,000 per year! By 2020 it is predicted that 13% of all deaths will be due to tobacco. The economic impact of tobacco consumption is not too good either. 9000 crore cigarettes smoked in a year cost Rs. 18,000 crore. Rs. 24,400 crore is the sale value of all tobacco products. And what is the results of these whopping statistics? We get 400,000 cancer cases annually and 1,300,000 cases of heart disease. We are world leaders in oral cancer and we spend 27,761 crores on treating tobacco-related diseases!

Those who smoke not only harm themselves but persons staying near them are also harmed by second hand smoke. Among children, sudden infant deaths, respiratory illnesses, middle ear disease, gum and tooth disease and Asthma are common due to this. Among the adults, lung cancer and heart diseases are well known.

9.1 Most Smokers would quit but . . .

Studies show that 75-85% of the smokers want to quit smoking. 1/3rd make a serious attempt to quit but only 1-2% are abstinent at the end of first year. Even a brief advice (lasting 3 minutes) by physician can improve quit rates. 70% of smokers visit a physician each year. Smokers cite physician advice to quit as an important motivator to quit. What do these data suggest? Smokers are interested in quitting, clinicians are frequently in contact with smokers and that they have a high credibility with the smokers. Unfortunately only 15% of smokers who visit a physician are offered some form of assistance and only 3% have a follow-up visit to address the issue even though physician's advice requires little in terms of money and time.

9.2 The 5 A's might help—National Cancer Institute says

For the patients who wish to stop there are 5 A's—for patients willing to quit, National Cancer Institute advices a 5 A-based intervention in a primary care. ASK, ADVISE, ASSESS, ASSIST and ARRANGE.

(i) "ASK"—All tobacco users identified at each visit.
(ii) "ADVICE" should be Clear, Strong and Personalized.
(iii) "ASSESS" the willingness to quit. Provide

motivational assistance.

(iv) "ASSIST"—Help the patient with a quit plan. Set a quit date within the next two weeks.

(v) "ARRANGE" for follow-up contact.

9.3 Psychosocial Approaches

Behaviour therapies include skills training and relapse prevention by identifying various causes which can lead to relapses and then learning how to deal with these situations. In aversive therapy, smoking is made aversive and less reinforcing by inducing mild nicotine intoxication symptoms of nausea and vomiting, etc. when the patient smokes (by rapid smoking). Other approaches can be self-help materials, educational and supportive groups, hypnosis, exercise, Biofeedback, family therapy, interpersonal therapy and Psychodynamic therapy have all been used for smoking cessation.

9.4 Medical Approach

Medication can be administered as replacement therapy, antagonist therapy, therapies to make drug intake aversive and non-nicotine medications that mimic nicotine effects. Non-medication somatic therapies include acupuncture and other devices.

(a) Nicotine Replacement Therapies (NRT's)

Nicotine Replacement Therapies (NRT's) are the appropriate first line agents. These are not to be used in heart patients such as immediate (2 wks) post-MI period, serious arrhythmias and serious or worsening angina pectoris. Use in pregnant and lactating women should be guarded. Nicotine chewing gum improves long-term abstinence rates by 30 to 80%. It is available as OTC in USA. For those smoking 1-25 cig., 2 mg gum and for > 25 cigs. a 4 mg gum per day is indicated. Duration of treatment is 12 weeks. Side effects are soreness and dyspepsia. Nicotine Patch, Nasal spray and Inhalers double smoking cessation rate. Duration of therapy is 6 months with dose tapering in last 3 months. Local irritation, cough and rhinitis are frequent side effects.

Writing for *The Tribune*, Chandigarh (Wednesday,

January 29, 2003) A.S. Prashar says, despite all efforts, the habit of smoking and tobacco chewing is spreading in the country like never before. Lakhs of tobacco users join the ranks of those already in the vice-like grip of this dangerous habit. And almost all the new recruits to their ranks are youth. Incidentally, smoking has become fashionable not only among young men but also among young women. And once they get hooked, it is difficult to kick the habit. The use of indigenous tobacco products like snuff, zarda, khaini and gutka has resulted in India recording the world's highest incidence of oral cancer. According to National Cancer Registry programme, it is estimated that annually 75,000-80,000 new oral cancer cases develop in India every year, of which 90 per cent can readily be attributed to the use of gutka and such other products.

Medical circles regard the incidence and growing rate of tobacco-related cancer as alarming. "A regular gutka consumer is not only unaware of the health hazards, but the addiction is severe and difficult to kick. With the absence of alternatives, he is left with no choice but to continue with the habit. While there are gutka bans in-effect, they can be ineffective unless a safe and healthy alternative is made available. Nicotine Replacement Therapy (NRTs) are that safe alternative, which have the added benefit of improving dental hygience among tobacco chewers"

NRT products have been available in the West for more than a decade, and are recommended by the World Health Organization (WHO) as the most safe and effective aid available to tobacco addicts seeking to quit their dangerous smoking and chewing habits. NRTs reduce, and in most cases eliminate, the withdrawal symptoms experienced by tobacco users by delivering a safe, pure, a regulated dose of nicotine. With the reduction or elimination of withdrawal symptoms, most tobacco users find quitting their tobacco habits much easier.

Ceejay Health Care Private Limited has become the first company outside the US to introduce India's first Nicotine Replacement Therapy (NRT) product, India's first safe and government approved answer to the carcinogenic smoking has now become available in the country. "Indians have often toyed with the idea of kicking the habit of gutka, cigarettes and tobacco chewing. Nicotine Replacement Therapy is a globally approved method of ending tobacco dependence. NuLife is India's first NRT and its first step towards eliminating tobacco addiction," says chairman of the company. Called NuLife Chewettes, they are chewing gums available in a proprietary, ethnic Indian "Good Kha" flavour for gutka chewers and a soon be released "Euco-Mint" flavour for smokers. They contain the pharmaceutical ingredient, nicotine polacrilex, widely used in the west as a safe and effective aid in tobacco cessation, and have none of the more than 4,000 carcinogens present in tobacco products such as cigarettes and gutka. "Tobacco addicts, especially gutka chewers, love the feel of chewing tobacco; hence we thought of a chewing gum substitute, which will give them the "chew" feel, the taste they like, without any of the harmful effects of gutka".

(b) Medication that Mimic Nicotine Effects

(i) Bupropion SR (a Non-nicotine medication with abstinence rate twice that of the placebo).
(ii) Clonidine.
(iii) Anxiolytics.
(iv) Antidepressants.
(v) Stimulants.
(vi) Anorectics.
(vii) Sensory Replacement—(Black pepper extracts, capsaicin, denicotinised tobacco, flavourings all decrease cigarette craving and withdrawals, a critic acid inhaler).
(viii) Acupuncture.

The various above mentioned methods have been used alone or in various combinations with mixed results, but ultimately it is the willingness/motivation of the patient which is of utmost importance in the matter of smoking cessation. Only when the patient is willing to stop smoking, the physician can help him. At the end the message is "Even single puff is detrimental to quit attempt."

10. MYTHS ABOUT SMOKING

10.1 Myth—I can quit smoking whenever I like

Nicotine is one of the most addictive substances on earth, and most people who try to quit cigarettes will have a hard time breaking its hold, according to the National Institute on Drug Abuse. The chemical goes directly from the lungs to the brain and stimulates the production of dopamine, a chemical that makes you feel happy. Although nicotine can make you feel more animated and energetic when you start smoking, your body will need more and more of it to feel the same way later on. If you do quit, you may find the craving to light up almost unbearable, and you're likely to get headaches and feel tired, sleepy, hungry, or irritable. In fact, 35 million people attempt to quit smoking every year, but only 7 percent of them actually succeed. But that doesn't mean you can't do it: 2.5 million people quit smoking every year. The most successful quitters use support groups, nicotine replacement therapy (gum or patches), or a combination of approaches. Many of them have to try more than once to quit altogether.

10.2 Myth—Smoking will hurt me alone, why bother

The dangers of second hand smoke are well documented. If you light up, you're exposing your children, spouse, and other family members to substances that can cause lung cancer, heart disease, asthma and other diseases. Second hand smoke kills an estimated 35,000 to 65,000 non-smokers each year. Up to 62,000 will die from heart disease, and about 3,000 will die from lung cancer, according to the National Cancer Institute. Tobacco smoke in the environment makes non-smokers more susceptible to ear infections, asthma attacks, and other respiratory problems, the Environmental Protection Agency reports. If you're pregnant and smoking, you run a higher risk of having a miscarriage or a stillborn infant, according to the U.S. Surgeon General. Your baby also runs a higher risk of dying from Sudden Infant Death Syndrome or SIDS, recent studies indicate. That's why one of the most important things you can do to ensure a safe pregnancy—along with avoiding alcohol and getting prenatal care—is to stop smoking.

10.3 Myth—Cigar smoking and chewing tobacco are safe

It's not only cigarette smoke that can kill you. Overall cancer death rates among men who smoke cigars are 34 percent higher than cancer death rates among non-smokers according to the American Lung Association. Cigar smokers have higher death rates from chronic obstructive pulmonary disease and are four to 10 times more likely to die from cancers of the throat, mouth, lips, larynx, and esophagus than non-smokers, the National Cancer Institute reports.

People who chew tobacco don't get off lightly either. If you chew tobacco, you're more likely to get oral cancer, which affects the tongue, lips, cheeks, and gums. Moreover, a 1995 study of 6,300 smokeless tobacco users reported in the *American Journal of Public Health* that they were twice as likely as non-users to die of heart disease.

As with cigarette smoking, the sooner you quit, the better your chance of escaping these diseases.

10.4 Myth—Smoking lowers blood pressure

No one knows where this one started, but many people believe that smoking or chewing tobacco actually helps them relax by lowering their blood pressure. This myth has no scientific merit. In 1998, a group of researchers in Stockholm, Sweden studied 135 healthy people who had never been diagnosed with high blood pressure. But after their blood pressure was measured, scientists found that those who smoked or chewed tobacco had higher pressure than those who didn't.

10.5 Myth—Smoking elevates mood

Some people believe smoking lifts the spirits, but it can sink your mood. If you're already down or depressed, cigarettes can put you at higher risk for clinical depression, hyperactivity, and attention deficit disorder, according to a recent report in the journal Pediatrics. Teens who smoke are four times as likely to be depressed as teens that don't, the study revealed.

10.6 Myth—I smoke only a few cigarettes, that is not harmful

Smoking isn't safe even if you're smoking one cigarette

a day. Every cigarette contains about 1 to 2 milligrams of nicotine, and it reaches your brain 10 seconds after you inhale. Immediately after that first puff, you'll get a rush of adrenaline that may increase your blood pressure, your heart rate, and your breathing.

10.7 Myth—I smoke safe, filtered cigarettes

Smokers who puff on only one or a few cigarettes a day or smoke low-tar cigarettes have a tendency to take more drags on the few cigarettes they allot themselves each day because they sense they're getting less nicotine and need to fill that craving. Despite the filters, nicotine and other dangerous chemicals still get through when you smoke. People who smoke filtered or low-tar brands may inhale even more deeply, thereby getting more carbon monoxide and other substances into their lungs, according to the National Cancer Institute.

10.8 Myth—Smoking causes only lung cancer and incidence of that is low

Unfortunately, this isn't the case. Smoking causes a number of other lung diseases, including emphysema, a degenerative disease that makes breathing more and more difficult. Smoking also increases your risk of heart disease, particularly if you have high blood pressure or high cholesterol, and aggravates many digestive disorders as well. It can also cause cancer of the mouth, larynx (voice box), and esophagus, according to the American Lung Association. Smoking also plays a role in cancer of the pancreas, kidney, bladder, and, in women, cancer of the cervix.

10.9 Myth—If I stop smoking, I will gain weight

It's true that many smokers gain weight once they stop smoking. Many of them substitute eating for the oral gratification that comes from puffing on a cigarette. On average, quitters again gain only 5 to 10 pounds. But once you've stopped smoking, the weight gain doesn't have to be permanent. In fact, if you exercise, you may not only lose the weight you've gained, and you may increase the stamina and lung capacity you lost when you were smoking. To help you keep the weight-off, replace smoking with other activities besides eating: chewing gum, doodling, sucking on a straw, or just stretching and breathing deeply.

For some people, the concern about gaining weight can be moderated with counseling—as can the weight gain itself. One study showed that women who were counseled about their concerns regarding weight gain after smoking cessation gained fewer pounds than those who weren't.

10.10 Myth—Smoking is cool and sexy

Smoking stains your teeth, causes wrinkles in your face, and puts cigarette burns in your clothes. It won't do wonders for your breath or your overall aroma, either. In one recent poll, 86 percent of teens said they'd rather date a non-smoker than a smoker. Moreover, studies show that men with high blood pressure who smoke are far more likely than non-smokers to become impotent. That's not exactly sexy.

And one last myth, perhaps the most important one of all.

10.11 Myth—I have smoked for years, even if I stop now, it will not help

If you smoke, you're cutting years off your life. A 35-year old man, for instance, will live about five years longer just by quitting smoking, according to the National Institute on Drug Abuse. The same holds true for women. The good news is that as soon as you stop smoking, you may not only begin to breathe easier, you may taste your food again, too. You can't turn back the clock, but if you quit smoking for a decade or more, your risk of cancer is much lower and your risk of heart disease may be almost the same as someone who's never smoked.

References

American Lung Association. Secondhand Smoke and Your Family. http://www.lungusa.org/tobacco/smosecondha.html

American Lung Association's Myths on Cigar, May 9, 1996. http://www>.lungusa.org/press/association/asscigarmyth.html

Bolinder, G. *et al.* American Journal of Hypertension. 1999 Sep; 12 (9 pt 1): 948-9 Ambulatory 24-hour blood pressure monitoring in healthy, middle-aged smokeless tobacco users, smokers, and non-tobacco users.

Bolinder, G. Smokeless tobacco use and increased cardiovascular mortality among Swedish construction workers. *American Journal of Public Health*, 1995 Jan; 85 (1): 118-19.

Centres for Disease Control and Prevention. Tobacco information and prevention sources: Facts you should know. November 2000.

Edwin B. Fisher Jr., PhD. 7 steps to a Smoke-Free Life, American Lung Association, John Wiley '& Sons Inc. 1998.

Goodman, Elizabeth, MD and John Capitman, PhD. Depressive Symptoms and Cigarette Smoking Among Teens. *Pediatrics*, 2000; 106: 748-55 October, 2000.

Jacobs, Edward A., MD, et al. Tobacco's Toll: Implications for the Pediatrician. Committee on Substance Abuse, 2000-2001, *Pediatrics*, 2001; 107: 794-98.

National Cancer Institute. Questions and Answers About Cigar Smoking and Cancer.

National Institute on Ageing. Smoking: It's Never Too Late to Stop. http://www.aoa.dhhs.gov/aoa/PAGES/AGEPAGES/smoking.html.

National Institute on Drug Abuse. Nicotine Addition. http://www.nida.nih.gov/ResearchReports/Nicotine/nicotine1.html#addictive

Smoking cessation and the course of major depression: a follow-up study. Glassmarr AH; Covey LS; Stener F; Rivelli S comment in Lancet. 2001 Jun 16; 357(9272): 1900-1, 21319304.

U.S. Surgeon General. "Women and smoking: A report of the Surgeon General—2001," www.cdc.gov/tobacco <http://www.cdc.gov/tobacco>/sgr/sgr_forwomen/ataglance.htm

Goodman, Elizabeth, MD and John Capitman, PhD. Depressive Symptoms and Cigarette Smoking Among Teens. *Pediatrics*, 2000; 106 : 748-55 October, 2000.

Smoking cessation and the course of major depression: a follow-up study. Glassman AH; Covey LS; Stetner F; Rivelli S comment in Lancet. 2001 Jun 16; 357 (9272): 1900-1, 21319304.

Jacobs, Edward A., MD, et al. Tobacco's Toll: Implications for the Pediatrician. Committee on Substance Abuse, 2000-2001, *Pediatrics*, 2001; 107 : 794-98.

IARC (International Agency for Research on Cancer). Tobacco smoking. Monographs on the evaluation of carcinogenic risk to Humans. Vol 38. Lyon: IARC, 1986.

Boyle P. Maisonneuve P. Lung cancer and tobacco smoking. *Lung Cancer*, 1995; 12:167-81.

Doll R, Peto R, Wheatley K, Gray R, Sutherland I. Mortality in relation to smoking: 40 years observation on male British doctors. *Br Med J*, 1994; 309: 901-11.

US Surgeon General: The health consequences of smoking: Cancer, Washington, DC, US Department of Health and Human Services.

Publ. No. 82-50179, 1982.

Behera D, Jindal SK, Malik SK. Primary adenocarcinoma of lung. Bull PGI. (Chandigarh). 1984; 18: 176-79.

Lubin JH, Li JY, Xuan XZ et al. Risk of lung cancer among cigarette and pipe smokers in Southern China. *Int J Cancer,* 1992; 51: 390-95.

Jindal SK, Behera D. Clinical spectrum of Primary lung cancer—review of Chandigarh experience of 10 years. *Lung India,* 1990; 8: 94-98.

Kaufman DW, Palmer JR, Rosenberg L *et al.* Tar content of cigarettes in relation to lung cancer. *Am J Epidemiol,* 1989; 129: 703-11.

Stockwell HG, Goldman AL, Lyman GH *et al.* Environmental tobacco smoke and lung cancer risk in nonsmoking women. *J Natl Cancer Inst,* 1992; 84 : 1417-22.

United States Environmental Protection Agency. Respiratory health effects of passive smoking: Lung cancer and other disorders. Office of Health and Environmental assessment; Office of Research and Development, U.S. Environmental Protection Agency, EPA/600/6-90/006F, December 1992.

Wynder EL. The aetiology, epidemiology, and prevention of lung cancer. *Semin Respir Med,* 1982; 3: 135.

Chia SE, Chia KS, Phoon WS, Lee HP. Silicosis and lung cancer among Chinese granite workers. Scand J. Jindal SK, Behera D. Clinical spectrum of Primary lung cancer—review of Chandigarh experience of 10 years. *Lung India,* 1990; 8: 94-98. *Work Environ Health,* 1991; 17: 170-74.

Burns PB, Swanson GM. The occupational cancer incidence surveillance study (OCISS): risk of lung cancer by usual occupation and industry in the Detroit metropolitan area. *Am J Ind Med,* 1991; 19: 655-71.

Jockel KH, Ahrens W, Wichmann HE, *et al.* Occupational and environmental hazards associated with lung cancer. *Int J Epidemiol,* 1992; 21: 202-13.

Karjalainen A, Anttila S, Vanhala E, Vainio H. Asbestos exposure and the risk of lung cancer in a general urban population. *Scand J work environ Health,* 1994; 20: 243-50.

Whitessell PL, Drage CW. Occupational lung cancer. *Mayo Clin Proc,* 1993; 68: 183-88.

Scali J, Astre C, Segala C, Gerber M. Relationship of serum cholesterol, dietary and plasma β-carotene with lung cancer in male smokers. *Eur J Cancer Prev,* 1995; 4: 169-74.

Alavanja MCR, Brown CC, Swanson C, Brownson RC. Saturated fat intake and lung cancer risk among non-smoking women in Missouri. *J Natl Cancer Inst,* 1993; 85: 1906-16.

Sideny S, Cann BJ, Friedman GD. Dietary intake of β-carotene in non-smokers with and without passive smoking at home. *A J Epidemiol,* 1989; 129: 1305-09.

Pastorino U, Pisani P, Berrino F *et al.* Vitamin A and female lung cancer: A case control study on plasma and diet. *Nutr cancer,* 1987; 10: 171-79.

World Health Organization. Cancer in developed countries: Assessing the trends. *WHO Chron*, 1985; 39: 109.

Khuri FS, Herbst RS, Fossells FV. Emerging therapies in non-small-cell lung cancer. *Ann Oncol*, 2001 12: 739-44.

Parkin DM, Muir CS, Whelan S, Gao YT, Ferlay J, Powell J, Editors. Cancer incidence in five continents, Volume VI, IARC Scientific Publication Number 120; Lyon, IARC, 1992.

Ferlay J, Bray F, Pisari P, Parkin DM. Cancer Incidence, mortality and prevalence world-wide. IARC, WHO, IARC Press, Lyon, 2001.

Hammond EC, Horn D. Smoking and death rates-Report on 44 months of follow up of 187, 783 men. II. Death rates by cause. JAMA; 1958: 166: 1294.

Parkin DM, Pisani P, Ferlay J. Estimates of the worldwide incidence of eighteen major cancers in 1985. *Int J Cancer*, 1993; 54: 594-606.

Negri E, La Vecchia C. Epidemiology of lung cancer: recent trends in mortality with emphasis on Europe. *Lung Cancer*, 1995; 12 (Suppl 1): S3—S11.

Viswanathan R., Gupta S, Iyer PVK. Incidence of primary lung cancer in India. *Thorax*, 1962; 17: 73-76.

National Cancer Registry Programme. Biennial Report, 1988-89. An Epidemiological study, Indian Council of Medical Research, New Delhi. Chapter 2. Cance Incidence. pp. 3-42.

Behera D, Kashyap S. Pattern of malignancy in a north Indian hospital. *J Indian Med Assoc.*, 1988 Feb; 86(2): 28-29.

Jindal SK, Behera D. Clinical spectrum of primary lung cancer—review of Chandigarh experience of 10 years. *Lung India*, 1990; 8: 94-98.

Gupta D, Boffetta P, Gaborieau V, Jindal SK. Risk factors of lung cancer in Chandigarh, India. *Indian J Med Res*, 2001 113: 142-50.

Gupta MP, Khanduja KL, Koul IB, Sharma RR. Effect of cigarette smoke inhalation on benzenepyrene induced lung carcinogenesis in Vitamin A deficiency in the rat. *Cancer Letter*, 1990; 55: 83-93.

Brown IM, Pottern LM, Blot WJ. Lung cancer in relation to pollutants emitted from industrial sources. *Environ Res*, 1984; 34: 250-61.

Wu JM, Du YX. Summary of papers and research recommendations presented at the International Symposium on lifestyle factors and human lung cancer, Guangzhou, China. Lung Cancer, 1996; 14 (Suppl 1): S223-S34.

Gao YT. Risk factors for lung cancer among nonsmokers with emphasis of lifestyle factors. *Lung Cancer*, 1996; 14 (Suppl 1): S39-S45.

Harris CC, Reddel R, Pfeifer A *et al*. Role of oncogenes and tumor suppressor genes in human lung carcinogenesis: In: O'Neil IKO, Chen J, Bartch, editors. Relevance to human cancer of nitroso compound, tobacco smoke, and mycotoxins. Lyons, International Agency for Research on Cancer. 1991; 294-303.

Carney DN. Oncogenes and genetic abnormalities in lung cancer. *Chest*, 1989; 96: 27S.

D. Behera, Professor Department of Chest Medicine, PGI. *Lung Cancer*, 2000. Edition 2002.

Clinical Practical Guidelines—Treating Tobacco Use and Dependence; US Department of Health and Human Services, Public Health Service.

The Health Benefit of Smoking Cessation—A report of the Surgeon General, 1990; US Department of Health and Human Services.

How to Stop Smoking—Rus LS and Maximin A; New Harbinger Publications Inc., 1997.

Cigarettes: What the Warning Label Doesn't Tell You—American Council on Science and Health; Magna Publishing Co., Mumbai, 2000.

6

CHANGES IN LIFESTYLE AND PREVENTION OF EYE DISEASE

JAGAT RAM* AND SUSHMITA KAUSHIK

INTRODUCTION

Changes in the lifestyle have been found to play major influence on occurrence and prevention of several human diseases such as diabetes mellitus, hypertension, allergic disorders, heart diseases and eye diseases. Nutrition and environmental intervention have been shown to be beneficial in preventing many eye diseases like cataract and age-related macular degeneration. A basic requisite of such beneficial intervention would be to bring about a change in lifestyle. Reviewed in this chapter are the eye diseases affected by external influences, and some simple lifestyle alterations that may prove beneficial in their prevention. By following the guidelines outlined below, we can help prevent and treat most of the eye diseases that occur with age, as well as maintain a healthier body and mind.

* Professor, Department of Ophthalmology, PGI, Chandigarh.

There are many factors that can contribute to the development of eye diseases. In addition to nutritional deficiencies, lifestyle choices such as smoking, alcohol consumption, lack of exercise, environmental conditions and stress can increase risks of ocular diseases. Heredity is also a leading factor in disease development.

I. NUTRITION AND OCULAR HEALTH

As the age-old saying goes, "Eat your carrots . . . they're good for your eyes!" Medical doctors and clinical scientists around the world have published numerous studies in leading medical journals about the preventive role nutrition can play in eye conditions, healing properties and diseases.[1,2] As we go through life, we tend to eat the same eight to twelve foods every week. But as our bodies change, so do our nutritional needs. Any nutritional deficiencies we may have in our daily diet can leave our eyes more vulnerable to sight-threatening diseases. In fact, the eyes are frequently the first part of the body to be affected by nutritional deficiencies.

What can be done?

Prevention and early detection are the keys in protecting vision. If the appearance of early signs of disease determines that one is at risk, specific measures may be recommended. Lifestyle changes such as exercising regularly, drinking plenty of water, minimizing alcohol consumption, not smoking and wearing UV protective sunglasses are all beneficial. Proper nutrition should be assured through a diet rich in anti-oxidants and if appropriate, nutritional supplements on a daily basis.

The Role of Free Radicals

Many eye disorders have been linked to "free radicals" which are formed when the body processes food and oxygen. Free radicals are unstable molecules that disrupt the structure of other molecules resulting in cellular damage within the eye.[3] As the body ages; it produces more free radicals while its ability to neutralize their negative effect decreases. Cancer, heart disease, stroke, and the major degenerative eye diseases—cataracts macular degeneration, glaucoma and diabetic retinopathy—are known to be caused, or at least exacerbated, by excess free radicals. Their pathogenesis can all be traced in large part to so-called "free radicals," reactive molecules that bombard our body on a daily basis both from inside and out. In fact, the aging process itself is believed by many scientists to be the sum total of all the destruction caused by these molecules. Through a process of oxidation (similar to rusting of metal), these free radicals have both good and bad effects.[4] On the one hand they help break down accumulated toxins, dead cells, and waste products in the body, and on the other hand they can damage healthy cells if not kept in control by our body's defense system.

To strengthen the body's defenses, nutritionists recommend increasing anti-oxidant levels through diet and nutritional supplements. Volumes of research prove that we can minimize (and reverse, in some cases) the damage that free radicals cause by reducing our exposure to them, by moderate exercise eating a more healthy diet, and by supplementing vitamins and minerals, especially the "anti-oxidants."[5]

Anti-oxidants are enzymes and nutrients that neutralize and deactivate free radicals. Those occurring naturally in the body or consumed in foods (Table 1) may block most of the damage. Over time, damaged cells can accumulate and lead to diseases such as macular degeneration, cataracts, glaucoma, diabetic retinopathy, and dry eye syndrome.[6] Increasing appropriate levels of anti-oxidants may be the most effective

Table 1

Vegetable and Fruits Rich in Anti-oxidants

Carrots	Onions
Garlic	Red & Purple Grapes
Cabbage	Pumpkin & Sunflower
Sweet Potatoes	Seeds
Green & Red	Strawberries
Pepper	Citrus Fruits
Spinach	Tomatoes
Broccoli	Green Tea
Cauliflower	

method of slowing or preventing this type of damage.

Dietary recommendations include eating five to nine servings of fresh fruits and vegetables each day while increasing our consumption of the good Omega 3 and 6 fats (found in vegetable oils, flax seed oil and fish oils, among others). Conversely, limiting sugar, saturated and "trans fat" (solid vegetable oils) consumption, and avoiding harmful chemicals such as aspartame (which is found in nearly all diet soft drinks—a substance may lead to massive chronic health complaints among baby boomers as we mature) and MSG (monosodium glutamate) due to their well documented toxicity. It's also essential to limit other chemical additives and carbonated beverages and it is recommended substituting filtered water and tea (esp. green tea) for soft drinks.

Why should we take Supplements?

Due to depletion of nutrients (especially minerals) in our farm soils it has been determined that even if we did eat a so-called "healthy" diet our food still lacks many of the essential micronutrients required to sustain optimum health. This does not mean that one will immediately become ill from nutritional deficiencies, as most problems show up only after many years. As we mature, our body becomes more and more susceptible to nutrient deficiency. Several studies have also shown that among older adults, those taking nutritional supplements reduced by half the number of ill days they experienced compared to a group of patients not taking supplements at all.[7]

Another reason supplements are essential to optimize our health is because in today's society we are exposed to many more toxins and more stress than at any time in history, while at the same time we are eating fewer fresh raw fruits and vegetables than ever before, many of which have much less nutritional value. These factors make it imperative to take nutritional supplements.

Recommended Doses

10-20,000 I.U. of mixed carotenoids (not just "beta" carotene, which has little benefit by itself) and Vitamin A, 500-1500 mg of Vitamin C, 200-800 I.U. of Vitamin E, and 200 mcg of Selenium (in the form of selenomethionine) are the recommended daily amounts of the most widely accepted anti-oxidants.[8] Vitamin C helps protect us from heart disease and boosts the immune system, while Vitamin E (400 I.U. to 800 I.U.) has been shown to reduce the risk of a second heart attack (the biggest killer in America) by as much as 77% in various peer reviewed studies. As far as the eyes are concerned, epidemiological studies of thousands of people showed that those with the lowest levels of these four nutrients were found to be 2.5X more likely to require cataract surgery. These anti-oxidants are just the starting point for a preventative approach to eye health. For maximum protection, a balanced supplement program is recommended, which includes B-Complex, amino acids, trace minerals (esp. chromium, magnesium and calcium), and phytonutrients, taken with meals in at least two daily doses. An effective program requires taking a minimum of five to six capsules daily to obtain adequate protection.

To summarize, controlling free radicals helps to minimize their negative impact on the degenerative eye diseases. A preventive approach toward ocular disease is beneficial, by starting before problems manifest themselves. This could be achieved by having regular eye examinations, getting exercise, eating well and by taking quality nutritional supplements on a daily basis.

2. THE EFFECT OF THE EXTERNAL ENVIRONMENT

The external environment affects the ocular surface most frequently. The main factors are dry and dusty environment, pollution, pollen, heat and sunlight. Major problems include dry eye, ocular allergy, and adverse effects of sunlight and ultraviolet (UV) radiation.

(a) Dry Eye

Dry eye syndrome is one of the most common problems treated by eye physicians. It is usually caused by a problem with the quality of the tear film that lubricates the eyes. In addition to lubricating the eye, tears are also produced as a reflex response to outside stimulus such as an injury or emotion. However, reflex tears do little to soothe a dry eye, which is why someone with watery eyes may still complain of irritation. Dry eye syndrome has many causes. One of the most common reasons for dryness is simply the normal aging process. As we grow older, our bodies produce less oil—60% less at age 65 than at age 18.

Many other factors, such as hot, dry or windy climates, high altitudes, air-conditioning and cigarette smoke also exacerbate dry eyes.[9] Many people also find their eyes become irritated when reading or working on a computer. Stopping periodically to rest and blink keeps the eyes more comfortable. Contact lens wearers may also suffer from dryness because the contacts absorb the tear film, causing proteins to form on the surface of the lens. Certain medications, thyroid conditions, Vitamin A deficiency, and diseases such as Parkinson's and Sjogren's can also cause dryness. Women frequently experience problems with dry eyes as they enter menopause because of hormonal changes.

Can Certain Fats Relieve Dry Eye Symptoms?

Recently, attention has been drawn to nutrition and its affect on the maintaining the body's balance of natural oils by supplementation of essential fatty acids (EFA). A deficiency of EFAs has been linked to many diseases and disorders. They are also believed to affect how the body's glands produce oil. Because of this, increasing the intake of EFAs may improve conditions such as dry eyes and dry skin. The body does not produce EFAs, so they must be supplied through diet. It is essential to consume EFAs properly for the body to receive their full benefit. The following is a suggested regimen:

- ❑ 12 almonds or pecans daily (Substituting peanuts for almonds and pecans will not produce the same result!)
- ❑ 3 evening primrose oil capsules (500 mg) 2 or 3 times daily.

There is no perfect cure for dry eye syndrome, but taking these simple steps, along with other treatments like lubricating eye drops, can give relief from the frustrating symptoms.

(b) Allergy

Allergic reactions are triggered by the body's immune system to protect the eyes from injury. The immune system mistakes usually harmless substances (such as pollens) for unwanted foreign intruders (such as bacteria) and overreacts, producing allergy symptoms ranging from mild to severe. The result can be considerable discomfort, tissue damage and sometimes, impaired vision.[10]

Allergic reactions in the eyes, known as allergic conjunctivitis, can result from a variety of causes. Some allergies are seasonal; others are perennial (affecting sufferers unpredictably throughout the year). Food sensitivities also can cause allergic reactions in the eyes.

Different types of eye allergies, many of which share common symptoms, include:

- ❑ Swelling of the eye area, or hives, usually due to food allergies.
- ❑ Itching of the eye area caused by contact with wool, climatic changes, excessive exposure to soap, water, oils and cosmetics.
- ❑ Inflammation, eye irritation and watering due to contact with an irritating substance.
- ❑ Inflammation of the cornea, resulting in eye pain, sensitivity to light, eye secretions and tearing.

Simply visiting an eye care professional may alleviate allergy-related eye problems.

Allergies and infections may exhibit the same symptoms. That's why self-diagnosis or treatment should be avoided, because it could make the condition worse. There are many options for relieving the misery of eye allergy symptoms.

Following are suggestions for relief:

- ❑ Cold compresses. "Dampen a washcloth with cold water. Then place it over your eye lids."
- ❑ Use non-prescription eye drops that combine

antihistamines and decongestants such as topical Naphazoline azelastine.

- For severe or persistent symptoms, prescription medications may be needed, such as steroid eye drops.
- Wear sunglasses. Glasses greatly decrease the exposure to pollen particles, dust and polluting gases on the eye.

(c) Sunlight and Ultraviolet Exposure

The sun emits three types of ultraviolet radiation (UV-A 320-400 nm; UV-B 290-320 nm; UV-C 100-290 nm) that are very harmful to the skin and damaging to eyes. Those changes may result in a cataract, a clouding of the lens. Furthermore, epidemiological studies have shown that the risk for certain types of cataracts increases with increased exposure to UV, especially UV-B.[11] Scientists also suspect that long-term UV exposure may damage the sensitive retina at the back of the eye, contributing to macular degeneration, a major cause of vision loss in people over age 55.[12]

UV exposure also may cause pterygium, a fleshy growth on the white of the eye that can extend into the cornea and block vision. A hospital-based case-control study conducted in Singapore found a significantly higher risk of apterygial in those participants with longer solar exposures calculated over a 5 and 10-year period.[13]

One study from Australia also points towards an increased risk for choroidal and ciliary body melanoma with solar exposure. The incidence of these tumors was found to be positively associated with time spent outdoors.[14] A special type of macular burn called the solar burn is seen on days of solar eclipses, when people view the eclipse unaided. It is caused due to the direct exposure of the fovea to ultraviolet radiation from the sun.[15]

In addition to vision loss, excessive exposure to UV radiation—especially from light reflected off sand, snow or pavement—can produce a burn on the surface of the eye called photokeratitis. It's painful, like sunburn on skin, but the effects usually last only a few days. Protecting eyes from ultraviolet light is prudent. One must wear sunglasses that block 100 percent of the sun's ultraviolet rays.

(d) Eyes and Cosmetics

Cosmetics and hair dyes may be detrimental to the ocular surface by causing irritation, allergy or even a toxic response. The following is a recommended list of precautions to be taken while being judicious in the use of cosmetics:

- Close eyes when applying loose powder.
- Discard products used near the eye, such as mascara, eye liner and shadow, after six months.
- Cover eyes when using hair spray. (Pump bottles are easier to aim than aerosols).
- Avoid mascaras with lash extenders, which may get into the eye and cause irritations.
- Use water-based liners and mascara; they are easier to remove.
- Never apply eye liner to the inside of the eyelids. It can block tear glands and reduce the eye's ability to fight infection.
- Remove eye makeup with eyes shut. Use a non-oily remover.
- Dyes can harm eyes or lids. Be careful when dying hair.
- Don't direct a hair dryer toward eyes. If you sit under a dryer, use moisturizing drops.
- Don't share your cosmetics

3. PROFESSIONAL HAZARDS

Our eyes are affected through life by many things such as emotional factors, stress and type of work. For instance, over 90 percent of accountants are nearsighted, but less than 10 percent of the farmers are. That's because accountants spend an extreme amount of time looking at information on their desks and computers, and farmers are usually looking out across the fields.[16]

(a) The Computer Professional/Near Work Executive

Reflections from the computer monitor screen are one of

the causes of Computer Vision Syndrome (CVS). Reflections reduce the contrast of the images on the screen, which makes it more difficult to see and contributes to eyestrain. The answer is to use an anti-reflective screen on the monitor. The best type of anti-reflective screen is one that's glass and not mesh. Anti-Reflective coatings on eyeglasses do not reduce screen reflections. Although anti-reflective coatings enable an eyeglass wearer to see better in many situations they do not affect the reflections in the computer screen.

Stopping periodically to rest and blink also helps to reduce the effects of strain and dry eye which are much more common with long hours of computer work. The eyes should not be focused in one place for a sustained period of time. Sustained contraction of the eyes can lead to a contraction of the upper body and neck.

(b) The Outdoor Worker

The professionals who works outdoors most of the time is more likely to be affected by environmental factors of dust, dry wind, pollution and exposure to sunlight, as discussed in the previous section. Judicious use of protective glasses, and frequent eyewashes with cold water may help in alleviating these problems.

(c) Industrial Workers

Industrial workers suffer eye disorders related to exposure to the particular agent they work with. Chemical injuries are particularly devastating, and due precautions including protective eyewear, clothing, etc. are required while handing these lethal agents. Workers at firecracker units are vulnerable to both thermal and chemical burns in addition to the possibilities of inadvertent blast injuries. Rigorous safety precautions must be strictly adhered to in order to prevent debilitating ocular injury.

(d) Radiation Hazards

Radiation may be ionizing or non-ionizing. The former are more dangerous as regards ocular health. Radiation produces cell damage by free radicals generated as a result of ionization of water. This results in DNA damage leading to transcriptional errors and altered protein synthesis. The eye is comprised of radiosensitive tissues like the lens, conjunctive and cornea, which are often the first to be affected. Inadvertent exposure may lead to radiation dermatitis, skin depigmentation, conjunctival congestion and scarring, dry eye, corneal edema, superficial keratitis, and radiation cataracts.[17]

Exposure to X-Rays of a pregnant woman in the first trimester may cause congenital cataracts in the fetus. Chronic exposure to infrared radiation by glass-blowers may result in cataract formation. Others vulnerable to radiation exposure include inadequately protected medical staff, patients on treatment for malignancies and workers at atomic energy plants.

Preventive methods include radiation protective glasses, which are able to reduce exposure to the lens by 90%.

4. SMOKING

The single most important lifestyle change one can make is to stop smoking. Smoking impairs the body's circulation, decreasing the efficiency of the retinal blood vessels. It increases the risk of developing macular degeneration by up to six times, and more than doubles the risk for cataracts,[18,19,20] not to mention the increased risk of heart disease, dementia and stroke.

In one of the first extensive studies of its kind, researchers reviewed data from more than 20,000 male doctors who were surveyed for seven or more years. The study found that men who smoked a pack or more per day had a 2- to 3-fold increased risk of macular degeneration. Even former smokers showed increased risk for years after they quit smoking. Researchers theorize that smoking affects the blood supply to the retina, where the macular is located.[21,22]

One study provides evidence for a significant dose-response relationship between smoking and lens optical density.[23] Their data indicated that smoking is directly related to age-related increases in lens optical density throughout life, and these increases persist even after smoking cessation. Another study[24] linked cancer incidence among the visually impaired, where it tended to be increased for most cancer types. However, the excess in lung cancer was most correlated to age-related macular degeneration, which is more common amongst smokers.

5. ALCOHOL

Alcohol consumption has been implicated in the pathogenesis of cataract in some, but not all analytical studies. One prospective study suggested that there was a possibility of alcohol consumption leading to a modest increase in the risk of posterior sub-capsular type of opacities.[25] Another proposed association is the effect of alcohol on optic nerve function. A study of a Cuban epidemic of optic neuropathy revealed that the strongest epidemiological associations were with heavy drinking of alcohol, smoking, missed meals and weight loss.[26]

6. DRUGS

Long-term corticosteroids uses have long been known to be associated with cataract and glaucoma.[27] The occurrence and magnitude of adrenal suppression has been the most extensively evaluated systemic side effect studied. Population-based and limited randomized trials suggest that low-medium doses of inhaled corticosteroids do not cause cataract or glaucoma.[28] However, topical steroids may have more potent side effects. In addition to the aforementioned risks of cataract and glaucoma, they also lower the local ocular surface immunity, making the eye more susceptible to infections.

Corticosteroids must always be used judiciously only on the prescription of an ophthalmologist. The rampant use in simple allergies must be avoided and any actual requirement must be administered for the minimum time period required and monitored regularly.

Other commonly prescribed over-the-counter drugs usually have preservatives like benzalkonium chloride or thiomersal. They are epitheliotoxic and predispose the user to dry eye like symptoms. All drugs must be used with caution, and injudicious dosing "for the patients' satisfaction" strictly avoided.

7. CONSANGUINEOUS MARRIAGES AND HEREDITARY EYE DISEASES

Consanguinity is a social norm amongst certain communities in India. It has been implicated as a risk factor for cataract and certain congenital malformations of the eye. A report from Andhra Pradesh on the incidence of congenital colobomas amongst children showed that 43% of parents were consanguineous and 19% had a positive family history.[29]

Tremendous advances in the molecular genetics of human diseases have been made in the past decade. Many genes responsible for inherited eye disease have been isolated and characterized, and the chromosomal location of a number of additional genes has been determined. Some of these diseases include Dominant corneal dystrophies, aniridia, Peters' Anomaly, Juvenile glaucoma, Non-syndromic cataract, Stargardt's disease and retinoblastoma.

In general, most of the current approaches to gene therapy are aimed at repair of the somatic cells of the particular tissue affected. Specific treatment of the diseased cells does not however affect the other cells of the body, which includes the germ cells. Since the germ-cell lines continue to carry the flawed copies of the gene, the disease may still be passed onto the offspring of the parent. Therefore, genetic counseling of parents assumes a more important role, where restriction of the natural family and probably adoption of children would be a wise lifestyle decision.

8. SEXUALLY TRANSMITTED DISEASES AND THEIR EFFECT ON THE EYE

Syphilis and AIDS[30] are the most common sexually transmitted diseases that may manifest with ocular abnormalities. In addition, gonococcal and chlamydial vaginal infections may result in ophthalmia neonatorum of the newborn baby. Healthy lifestyle choices to prevent these diseases would include avoidance of promiscuity and adoption of safe sex methods like regular use of condoms.

How can Lifestyle Alterations Help Prevent Eye Disease?

Eye care in most countries is symptom-oriented. Ophthalmologists usually believe once something goes wrong with our eyes; there is not much that can be done in terms of reversing the process. Patients are taught hardly anything about prevention of problems. If people live long enough, severe visual impairment or blindness is almost inevitable. The eyes are particularly vulnerable to the effects of aging. Degenerative changes in the eye often begin in middle age. By age 70, a significant percentage of people suffer from macular degeneration, glaucoma and/or cataract. Diabetic retinopathy is also a major cause of visual disability among adults.

A review of the published scientific literature shows that common ocular disorders can be prevented with lifestyle changes. A compelling body of evidence indicates that orally ingested anti-oxidants and anti-glycating agents (such as carnosine) help to prevent and treat eye disease. Unfortunately, the aging process causes reduced blood flow to the eye. thereby inhibiting the delivery of orally ingested supplements into the eye.

Presented here are some benefits of changes in lifestyle in these three common ocular diseases of adulthood, viz. cataract, age-related macular degeneration, glaucoma and diabetic retinopathy.

(a) Cataract

It is estimated that 20 million people worldwide suffer from cataracts.[31] Many factors influence vision and cataract development such as age, nutrition, medications, smoking and sunlight exposure. High blood pressure, kidney disease, diabetes or direct trauma to the eye can also cause cataracts.

The aging process itself lends to certain metabolic changes that may predispose the lens to cataract development. Some of this occurs due to low supply of oxygen and nutrients, which leave the eye open to free radical damage. According to a 1983 report from the National Academy of Science, cataracts are initiated by free-radical hydrogen peroxide found in the aqueous humor. Free radicals such as hydrogen peroxide oxidize glutathione (GSH), destroy the energy-producing system of the eye, and allow leakage of sodium into the lens.[32] Water follows the sodium, and the edema phase of the cataract begins. Then, body heat in the lens of the eye oxidizes (cooks) lens protein, and it becomes opaque and insoluble (similar to egg protein).[33]

A lot of published research shows that the cataract progression can be slowed or prevented by the use of natural therapies and minor lifestyle changes.[34] Researchers at Harvard Medical School reported that oxidative mechanisms may play an important role in the pathogenesis of cataract and age-related macular degeneration, the two most important causes of visual impairment in older adults.[35] Preserving lens function through adequate anti-oxidant levels and delaying cataract formation by 10 years would result in saving at least half of the $3.2 billion spent annually in cataract surgeries and physician visits.[36]

Although it is difficult to treat cataracts with oral anti-oxidants since there is only minimal blood circulation within the eye compared to other parts of the body, nutritional supplements have been shown to reduce the risks of cataracts as well as slow or' reverse their progression. Results of a study[37] recently reported that plasma anti-oxidant levels influenced cataract development, independently of age, gender and other risk factors. Results showed that the risk of nuclear, cortical and posterior sub-capsular cataracts was lowest in individuals with the highest blood concentrations of carotene and beta-carotene, lycopene and lutein, respectively.

While the exact role of individual nutrients and optimum means of delivery (i.e., oral *vs.* topical) is not yet known, it has been demonstrated that anti-oxidants such as ascorbate, carotenoids and tocopherol, may protect against cataract formation.[38] A five-year study of over 3000 Wisconsin residents, aged 43 to 86, showed that the five-year risk for cataract was 60% lower among people who reported taking multi-vitamins or any supplement containing vitamin C or E on a long-term basis (more than 10 years) compared to non-users.[39] Similarly, a survey-based Harvard study of nearly 40,000 men aged 45 to 75 established, at eight-year follow-up, a 19% lower risk of cataract among men in the highest fifth of lutein and zeaxanthin intake compared to men in the lowest quintile.[40]

(b) Age-related Macular Degeneration (AMD)

Age-related macular degeneration (AMD) is the leading cause of blindness in people over the age of 55, affecting more than 10 million Americans. The incidence is high in India as well. Macular degeneration affects more Americans than cataracts and glaucoma combined. There are two forms of macular degeneration: atrophic (dry) and exudative (wet). Approximately 85% to 90% of the cases are the dry type. Both forms of the disease may affect both eyes simultaneously.

There is little that can be done within conventional medical treatment protocols to restore lost eyesight with either form of the disease. Leading researchers, however, are documenting the benefits of a more holistic approach in the treatment of AMD. Patients are encouraged to increase physical fitness, improve nutrition (including a reduction in saturated fats), abstain from smoking and protect their eyes from excessive light. Dietary supplementation of trace elements, anti-oxidants and vitamins is recommended for improving overall metabolic and vascular functioning. Early screening and patient education offer the most hope for reducing the debilitating effects of the disease.

Exposure to light and photochemical damage have been suspected factors in AMD as well as decreased anti-oxidant activity responsible for damage control.[41] An age-dependent drop in glutathione blood status, and a significantly lower level of glutathione has been found in older individuals compared to younger ones. Moreover, an increase of oxidized glutathione by-product over time suggests more oxidation and the incumbent higher risk of age-related eye diseases.[42] Glutathione, which is particularly concentrated in the lens, has been shown to have a hydroxyl radical-scavenging function in lens epithelial cells.

Lutein and zeanxanthin, the primary carotenoids concentrated in the macula, counter the free-radical forming action of light and oxygen. It has been suggested that the macular pigment protects the retina via a dual role that includes scavenging for free radicals and filtering out blue light, which can cause photochemical damage.[43] Some studies have also suggested a link between dietary carotenoid intake and macular pigment density. Eyes with age-related maculopathy (ARM) have revealed significantly lower carotenoid and ascorbate levels in the macula and retina than healthy eyes.[44]

(c) Glaucoma

Glaucoma, usually an inherited disease, results from the build-up of intraocular pressure. Generally, the condition develops after age 40, although congenital glaucoma and physical injury to the eye can account for earlier age of onset. Figures show that 1 out of every 25 Americans suffers from glaucoma, and over 62,000 are legally blind due to glaucoma. Age-related losses of anti-oxidants increase physical stress on the eye, and oxidative damage ensues. Diminished anti-oxidant activity in lacrimal (tear) fluid and blood plasma seems to coincide with progression of glaucoma.

Medications often have side effects, and rarely correct the cause of the patient's problems. The first treatment step in non-acute glaucoma cases should be to evaluate the patient's lifestyle regarding management of stress, emotional factors, diet and exercise. The second step is to provide a nutritional supplementation program to include those nutrients shown in studies to be missing in people with specific conditions.[45] In the case of glaucoma, these nutrients include alpha lipoic acid and essential fatty acids.

There is evidence slowly mounting to support the effectiveness of various neuroprotective compounds in glaucoma.[46] A Russian study of 64 patients with primary open-angle glaucoma found that a combined regimen of hyperbaric oxygen and anti-oxidants over a five-year period stabilized visual function in 80% of patients.[47]

(d) Diabetic Retinopathy

One of the leading complications associated with diabetes is diabetic retinopathy steming from vascular damage. The damage causes the ruptured vessels to leak fluid, restricting oxygen and blurring sight, resulting in macular edema. As the disease progresses, the neovascularization on the surface of the retina results in proliferative diabetic retinopathy. The vitreous is composed of a fine network of hyaluronan gel, collagen, proteoglycans and fibronectin, all of which are susceptible to free radical damage brought on by light and UV damage and glycation.

Protein glycation occurs when sugar molecules inappropriately bind to protein molecules, forming cross-links that distort the proteins. Glycation appears to increase oxidative processes, which may explain why both glycation and oxidation simultaneously increase with age. High blood sugar also increases glycation activity, which may also explain the various kinds of tissue damage that characterize advanced diabetes.

Diligently controlling blood sugar is a major means of preventing or at least slowing the onset and progression of diabetic retinopathy. Researchers have found that diabetic patients who are able to maintain appropriate blood sugar levels have fewer eye problems than those with poor control. Diet and exercise play important roles in the overall health of those with diabetes. Diabetics can also greatly reduce the possibilities of eye complications by scheduling routine examinations with an ophthalmologist. Many problems can be treated with much greater success when caught early.

CONCLUSIONS: TIPS

To conclude, here are some tips on lifestyle changes, which may result in better ocular health, and prevention of degenerative ocular diseases:

1. Don't keep eyes focused in one place for a sustained period of time. Change focus; look up out of a window when doing near work.
2. Remember to wear UV-protective sunglasses to protect your eyes from the damaging effects of sunrays.
3. Quit smoking! Smokers have a significantly higher risk of eye disease than non-smokers.
4. Reduce sugar and alcohol intake. Do things in moderation.

Notes and References

1. Richer S. Nutritional influences on eye health. *Optometry*, 2000, Oct. 7-1(10):657-66.
2. Congdon NG, West KP Jr. Nutrition and the eye. *Curr Opin Ophthalmol*, 1999; 10:464-73.
3. Mares-Perlman JA, Klein R, Klein BE, Greger JL, Brady WE, Palta M, Ritter LL. Association of zinc and anti-oxidant nutrients with age-related maculopathy. *Arch Ophthalmol*, 1996; 114(8):991-7.
4. Beatty S, Koh HH, Henson D, Boulton M. The role of oxidant stress in the pathogenesis of age-related macular degeneration. *Surv Ophthalmol*, 2000; 45: 115.
5. Cai J, Nelson KC, Wu M, Steinberg P Jr. Jones DP. Oxidative damage and protection of the RPE. *Prog Retin Eye Res*, 2000, 19:205-21.
6. Richer OD. Anti-oxidants and the eye. *Int Ophthalmol Clin*, 2000; 40:1-16.
7. Carr AC, Frei B. Toward a new recommended dietary allowance for Vitamin C based on anti-oxidant and health effects in humans. *Am J Clin Nutr*, 1999; 69:1086-87.
8. Kaminski MS Yolton DP, Jordan WT, Yolton RL. Evaluation of dietary anti-oxidant levels and supplementation with ICAPS-Plus and Ocuvite. *J Am Optom Assoc*, 1993; 64:862.
9. Shimmura 5, Shimazaki J, Tsubota K. Results of a population-based questionnaire on the symptoms and lifestyles associated with dry eye. *Cornea*, 1999; 18408-11.
10. Allansmith MR. The eye and immunology. St. Louis:CV Mosby; 1982-75-81.
11. Taylor H, West SK, Rosenthal FS *et al*. Effect of ultraviolet radiation on cataract formation. *N Engl J Med.*, 1988; 319:1429-33.
12. Miller D. Clinical light damage to the eye. New York: Springer-Verlag; 1987.
13. Saw SM, Banerjee K, Tan D. Risk factors for the development of pterygium in Singapore: a hospital-based case-control study. *Acta Ophthlamol Scand*, 2000; 78:21 6-20.
14. Lerman S. Radiant energy and the eye. New York. MacMillan; 1980.
15. Vajdic CM, Kricker A, Giblin M, *et al*. Sun exposure predicts risk of ocular melanoma in Australia. *Int J Cancer* 2002; 10:175-82.
16. Cordain L, Eaton SB, Brand Miller J, *et al*. An evolutionary analysis of the etiology and pathogenesis of juvenile-onset myopia. *Acta Ophthalmol Scand*, 2002; 80:125
17. Merriam JR Szechter A, Focht EF. The effect of ionizing radiations on the eye. *Front Radiat Ther Oncol*, 1972; 6:346-85.
18. Harding JJ, Van Heyningen R. Risk Factors for cataracts. *Br J Ophthalmol*, 1989; 73:579-80.
19. Harding JJ. Cataract epidemiology. *Curr Opin Ophthalmol*, 1990; 1:10-15.

20. Hodge WG, Whitcher JP, Satarianow. Risk factors for age related cataract. *Epid Reviews*, 1995; 17:336-46.
21. The Eye Disease Case Control Study Group. Risk factors for neovascular age-related macular degeneration. *Arch Ophthalmol*, 1992; 110:1701-8.
22. Seddon JM, Hanankinson 5, Speizer F, Willert WC. A prospective study of cigarette smoking and age-related macular degeneration in women. *JAMA*, 1996; 276: 1141-6.
23. Hammond BR Wooten BR, Nanez JE, Wenzel AJ. Smoking and lens optical density. *Ophthalmic Physiol Opt*, 1999; 19:3005.
24. Pukkana E, Verkasato PK, Ojarno M, *et al.* Visual impairment and cancer: a population-based cohort study in Finland. *Cancer Causes Control*, 1999; 10:13-20.
25. Chasan-Taber L, Willett WC, Seddon JM, Stampfer MJ, Rosner B, Colditz GA, Speizer FE, Hankinson SE. A prospective study of alcohol consumption and cataract extraction among U.S. women. *Ann Epidemiol*, 2000; 10:347-53.
26. Roman GC. An epidemic in Cuba of optic neuropathy, sensori-neural deafness, peripheral sensory neuropathy and dorsolateral myeloneuropathy. *J Neurol Sci*, 1994; 127:11-28.
27. Urban RC, Cotlier E. Corticosteroid-induced cataracts. *Surv Ophthalmol*, 1986; 31:102-10.
28. Sorkness CA. Establishing a therapeutic index for the inhaled corticosteroids. Comparisons of systemic activity and safety among different inhaled corticosteroids. *J Allergy Clin Immunol*, 1998; 102:552-64.
29. Hornby SJ, Ward SJ, ilbert CE, *et al.* Environmental risk factors in congenital malformations of the eye. *Ann Trop Paediatr*, 2002; 22:67-77.
30. Dugel PU, Rao NA. Ocular infections in acquired immune deficiency syndrome. *Int Ophthalmol Clin*, 1993; 33:103-27.
31. Thylefors B, Negrel AD, Parajasegaram R. Global data on blindness. *Bull WHO*, 1995; 73:115-21.
32. Benedek GB, Chylack LT, Libondi T *et al.* Quantitative determination of the molecular changes associated with early cataractogenesis in the living human lens using quazilastic light scattering. *Curr Eye Res*, 1987; 6:1421-32.
33. Ramalho JS, Marques C, Pereira PC, Mota MC. Role of glycation in human lens protein structure damage. *Eur J Ophthalmol*, 1996; 6:155-61.
34. Congdon NG. Prevention strategies for age related cataract: present limitations and future possibilities. *Br J Ophthalmol*, 2001; 85:516-20.
35. Delcourt C., Cristol JP, Leger CL, *et al.* Associations of anti-oxidant enzymes with cataract and age-related macular degeneration. *Ophthalmology*, 1999; 106:215-22.
36. Wu SY, Leske MC. Anti-oxidants and cataract formation: a summary review. *Int Ophthalmol Clin*, 2000 Fall; 40(4):71-81.
37. Cumming RG, Mitchell P, Smith W. Diet and cataract: the Blue Mountains Eye Study : *Ophthalmology*, 2000: 107:450-6.

38. Taylor A, Jacques PF, Chylack LT Jr, Hankinson SE, Khu PM, Rogers G, Friend J, Tung W, Wolfe JK, Padhye N, Willett WC. Long-term intake of vitamins and carotenoids and odds of early age-related cortical and posterior subcapsular lens opacities. *Am J Clin Nutr,* 2002; 75:540-9.
39. Mares-Perlman JA, *et al. Arch Ophthalmol,* 2000; 118:1556-63.
40. Brown L, et al. Am J Clin Nutr 1999; 70(4):517-524.
41. Goldberg J, Flowerdew G, Smith E, *et al.* Factors associated with age-related macular degeneration. An analysis of data from the first National health and nutritional examination survey. *Am J Epidemiol,* 1988; 128:700-10.
42. Cohen SM, Olin KL, Fever WJ *et al.* Low glutathione reductase and peroxidase activity in age-related macular degeneration. *Br J Ophthalmol,* 1994; 78:791-94.
43. Gerster H. Review: Anti-oxidant protection of the aging macula. *Age Aging,* 1991; 112:60-69.
44. Frei B, England L, Ames BN. Ascorbate is an outstanding anti-oxidant in human blood plasma. *Proc Natl Sci,* USA, 1989; 86:6377-81.
45. Stewart WC. The effect of lifestyle on the relative risk to develop open-angle glaucoma. *Curr Opin Ophthalmol,* 1995; 6:3-9.
46. Caprioli J. Neuroprotection of the optic nerve in glaucoma. *Acta Ophthalmol Scand,* 1997; 75:363-7.
47. Popova ZS, *et al.* Vestn Oftalmol, 1996 Jan; 112(1):4-6.

7

PREVENT CANCER: CONSUME SUITABLE NUTRIENTS (CHEMOPREVENTION)

K.L. KHANDUJA*

WHAT IS CHEMOPREVENTION AND HOW DOES IT WORK?

Chemoprevention is the attempt to use natural and synthetic compounds to intervene in the early stages of cancer, before invasive disease begins. This strategy is involved in the process of *carcinogenesis*—the transformation of a normal cell into a cancer cell. Currently, the National Cancer Institute, USA has made chemoprevention research a top priority; more than 400 potential agents are currently under investigation. Chemopreventive agents can act in two ways: they can prevent or stop genetic mutations that lead to cancer, and they can prevent or stop processes that lead to excessive replication of damaged cells. Chemoprevention should not be confused with chemotherapy. Chemotherapy's aim is to kill cells, particularly cancer cells, in the hope of preventing further

* Professor and Head, Department of Biophysics, PGI, Chandigrh.

cancer progression. Chemoprevention, on the other hand, involves administering non-toxic agents to otherwise healthy individuals who may be at increased risk for cancer.

NATURAL GIFTS

Food is a source of some of the most exciting chemopreventative research. Epidemiological studies show that people with diets high in fruits and vegetables have lower risk for many types of cancers. However, trying to isolate individual chemicals within the food for cancer prevention has been very difficult. One well-studied example is beta-carotene. Once dubbed a strong cancer preventative, the supplement has been shown to actually increase the risk of lung cancer in adults who smoke tobacco.

As yet, we are unsure what part of the fruits and vegetables are protective. Perhaps it is the combination of various substances within whole fruits and vegetables and which cannot be reduced down into a simple supplement. Perhaps as 'nature made it' is best

CHEMOPREVENTION—THE ANSWER TO CANCER?

Recently, you may have heard the words *chemoprevention*, *nutraceuticals*, and *phytochemicals* in the media. What exactly do these terms mean? With the ever-increasing interest in improving our health, it is important to understand these words and understand their function in health care. The information presented here will provide a basis for deciphering the mixed messages that are being delivered in the media, conversations, research and education.

Research has demonstrated that cancer is a largely avoidable disease. It is estimated that more than two-thirds of cancer may be prevented through lifestyle modification: (1) Nearly one-third of these cancer occurrences can be attributed to diet alone, secondary to diet of high-fat, low-fiber content. Fruit and vegetable consumption have been consistently shown to reduce the risk of many cancers; (2) A major prevention strategy has been the program sponsored by the various Health Agencies, encouraging the public to include more fruits and vegetables in their diet. The following guidelines have been developed for the better health:

- Choose most of the foods you eat from plant sources.
- Limit your intake of high-fat foods, particularly from animal sources.
- Be physically active. Achieve and maintain a healthy weight.
- Limit consumption of alcoholic beverages if you drink at all.

Consequently, even before these guidelines were developed, researchers began investigating several substances that have the potential to inhibit cancer tumor formation. This investigation evolved into what is called "chemoprevention" today. The "chemoprevention" strategy of preventing cancer was founded in the mid-1970s by Michael B. Sporn, an innovator in cancer prevention research. Successful trials involving chemopreventive agents and animals led scientists to design larger similar trials with humans.

ANTI-OXIDANTS

As the name implies, an anti-oxidant protects the body from the effects of oxidation from oxygen. During the normal process of converting nutrients to energy (called metabolism), the body creates free radicals; they also enter the body through toxins in foods. Free radicals are atoms with an unpaired electron which easily combine with other molecules in the body causing random chemical reactions (oxidation). If the formation of free radicals is left unchecked, the effects of oxidation can accumulate over time and damage the body in various ways. This damage from oxidation has been associated with signs of aging and with chronic degenerative diseases such as arthritis, heart disease, and cancer. One of the primary ways that the healthy body intercepts free radicals before they do any damage is with anti-oxidants, which 'mop up' or neutralize free radicals so that they can no longer cause damaging chemical reactions. Presumably, lycopene, among other free radical scavengers, if present in adequate amounts, can help protect the body against free radical damage. Studies have shown that lycopene is more than twice as effective as beta-carotene.

Free radicals are caused by the living pocess of burning our food and by contaminates [carcinogens] in our bodies. The cleaner the burning process the fewer the free radicals, but all living creates free radicals. Well trained athletes for example step up their anti-oxidant intake before and after strenous exercises to neutralize the free radicals given off by the exercise. Vitamin C is an anti-oxidant working in the fluids that surround the cell. Vitamin E is fat soluble and works inside the cell. These anti-oxidants must be in place in sufficient quantities at all times to lower the free radical damage. Other anti-oxidants also help and many are even more powerful than the two vitamins mentioned, but the body needs both the fat soluble and water soluble anti-oxidants. Flax seed oil, Evening primrose, Vitamin A, Beta carotene, and fish oils are good fat soluble sources. Vitamin C, Grape seed extract and melatonin are good water soluble sources. This all helps *prevent* cancer. The anti-Vitamin C crowd assumes that Vitamin C is for nutritional functions only and dismisses the anti-oxidant properties. They point out that Dr. Linus Pauling, who started the Vitamin C fad, died of cancer and so did his wife. What they fail to mention is that both were in their high 90's at death and had kept their cancers at bay for over 40 years.

Anti-oxidants are for prevention. Once the cancer has begun then the doctors step in to destroy the tumors. But free radical damage is happening at all times, and every day new cancerous cells are formed in every body, though for the most part the body destroys them. It is the *body's own* immune system that destroys these mutations. If more mutations happen than the immune system can handle, then tumors begin and we call this condition cancer. So if we keep the balance in our favour by lowering the incidence of mutations and helping to keep the immune system 'up to speed', the cancers can be kept at bay. Some anti-oxidants commonly used in cancer prevention and treatment are; Vitamin A and beta-carotene Vitamin C, Vitamin E, Zinc, Green Tea, Grape Seed Extract, Selenium, Coenzyme Q10, Cysteine, Gingko Biloba

ANTI-OXIDANT VITAMINS—ARE THEY CANCER-FIGHTERS?

Eating the vegetables and fruits that contains Vitamin E, C, and A, beta-carotene and Folic acid, as well as other protective substances, does appear to lower the risk for most cancers. This has been confirmed in study after study, which show, in general, that people whose diets are low in fruits and vegetables experience twice the risk of those with high intake. It is believed that there are a number of reasons for this. First, consuming generous quantities of fruits and vegetables generally replaces eating large amounts of animal fats. Studies have found high rates of many cancers in countries where consumption of animal fat is also high. The second important cancer-fighting property of vegetables and fruits is fiber, which is particularly effective against colon and rectal cancers. Third, most fruits and vegetables contain not only the valuable anti-oxidant vitamins but also important compounds known as phytochemicals. (Phyto comes from the Greek word for plant). These compounds fight cancer in a number of different ways. Some, such as the carotenoids and flavonoids, serve as anti-oxidants. Although dark green and yellow-orange vegetables are usually recommended for their abundance of carotenoids, one recent study has found that the carotenoid lycopene, a pigment that is responsible for the colour of tomatoes and other red fruits and vegetables, is a very potent anti-oxidant and may protect against colon and bladder cancer. Flavonoids are present in onions, apples, and wine. The phytochemical limonene, found in the peels of citrus fruits, blocks a protein that stimulates cell growth and proliferation and may inhibit a type of carcinogenic protein from entering healthy cells. Another important phytochemical under investigation is genistein, which is found in soy products. This substance helps to block estrogen and so, theoretically, might play a role in preventing breast cancer.

Experts advise eating five to nine servings of vegetables and fruits a day. In addition to vitamins, there are many complex phytochemical agents in fruits and vegetables that may not be cancer-protective individually but that may act together to produce benefits.

So what about those vitamin supplements? People at high risk for cancer, such as smokers, may want to take supplements of Vitamin E, which is not easily obtained in the diet. Taking a multiple vitamin, folic acid, and some extra Vitamin C probably won't hurt either. But the fact is, the path to health is lined with delicious, succulent fruits and vegetables, and eating them is much more fun than simply popping pills.

Researchers in the field of cancer and it's relationship to nutrition, published findings in Feb. 1999 which discusses the consistently lower risk of cancer for a variety of anatomic sites that is associated with higher consumption of tomatoes and tomato-based products and also with consumption of cruciferous vegetables, which he postulates may add further support for current dietary recommendations to increase fruit and vegetable consumption. However, the benefits derived from the lycopene in tomatoes has not yet been shown to profer an advantage to bladder cancer patients, though there has been an advantage observed for those with prostate cancer. Given that that prostate involvement is not uncommon with invasive bladder cancer, eating more tomato sauce products is a simple form of prevention worth considering.

Men of southern European descent, from regions where tomato-based foods are consumed more frequently (as part of the well-publicized "Mediterranean diet"), have a lower incidence of prostate cancer than African-American or Asian-American men who, typically, eat fewer tomato-based items. Even a pre-existing family history of prostate cancer did not change lycopene's protective effect, researchers' report. Lycopene from tomato juice is not easily absorbed, but when it's cooked with oil (as in making a sauce), this substantially increases intestinal absorption of its nutrients. In other words, cooked tomato sauce is a more efficient way of delivering lycopene to the body than raw tomato juice, according to this study. Researchers declared that, based on a mini-study of blood samples and dietary patterns of 121 men, those who consumed the most tomato sauce were the most likely to have high blood levels of lycopene. Consuming tomato sauce cooked with oil raised the blood level of lycopene by a factor of 2 to 3 times, as measured 24 hours after consumption; in comparison, uncooked tomato juice produced no measurable increase. However, lycopene from raw tomatoes may be able to protect against gastrointestinal cancers.

Lycopene is the predominant carotenoid found in the blood, in various tissues (such as liver, kidney, adrenal glands, testes, and ovaries), and in the prostate gland itself. Research suggests that lycopene is an essential part of the body's natural defense against harmful oxidizing agents such as free radicals. Lycopene is now being touted as a highly capable anti-oxidant. Researchers have now found that cooking carrots increases their anti-oxidant content by 34 percent. In fact, storing them for a week or two only increased their potency. This is similar to the observations concerning lycopene, the active anti-oxidant in tomatoes.

Many consumers think that fresh vegetables are always superior in nutritional quality than processed vegetables but this does not appear to be true for carrots. Leaving the carrots unpeeled is another way of increasing their anti-oxidant power. "Numerous phenolic compounds are located in the skin of fruits and vegetables, many of which are removed by peeling steps prior to processing," he notes. Cooking and storing breaks down the tough cell walls of the vegetables and frees the phenolic compounds that provide most of their anti-oxidant power.

GENESTEIN

A recent US study stated that the Asian diet, particulary the role of the phytochemical genestein-found in soy products—plays a direct role in Asia's lower incidence of invasive bladder cancer; "A significantly higher dietary consumption of soy products exists in Asia and has led to the notion that the isoflavones present in this diet may contribute to a reduction in the number of invasive transitional cell bladder cancers.

AGENTS MOST COMMONLY USED IN CHEMOPREVENTION

An agent must have minimal short-term and no known long-term toxicity. It must be highly effective, easy to administer, and be inexpensive. Food, a readily available item, contains several promising chemopreventive compounds such as certain vitamins, minerals, and phytochemicals. See the table below to find out more about these agents.

Agent	*Agent type*	*Cancer prevention/treatment*
Vitamin A + other retinoids	vitamin	skin, head + neck and lung
Vitamin C	vitamin	colon & stomach
Vitamin D	vitamin	colon
Vitamin E	vitamin	lung, head + neck, colon and stomach
Folic Acid	vitamin	pre-cancerous cells of the cervix
Selenium	mineral	skin
Calcium	mineral	colon
Beta-Carotene	phytochemical	lung, head + neck, colon & stomach
Monoterpenes	phytochemical	breast
Tamoxifen	drug	breast
Finasteride	drug	prostate
Oltipraz	drug	liver
NSAIDS (non-steroidal anti-inflammatory drugs—aspirin, buprofen)	drug	colon
Sunscreen	other	skin
Spirulina fusiformi	(blue-green algae)	other head + neck

IS CHEMOPROTECTION JUST A DREAM?

Progress in Chemopreventive Drug Development: Several hundred agents are at various stages of preclinical development.

Successes

In China and Japan, many epidemiological studies have found that tea drinkers have a lower than average incidence of cancer. Over the past decade, studies from other parts of the world have supported this conclusion. In a study involving 35,000 women in Iowa, those who drank at least two cups of tea a day had **60% less kidney and bladder cancer** and 32% less cancer of the esophagus and colon. A 15-year study of men in the Netherlands concluded that those who drank more than four cups of green tea a day were 69% less likely than others to suffer a stroke.

Some bacteria seem susceptible to catechins as well. Asian studies have shown that green tea inhibits bad breath, gum disease and tooth decay in laboratory rats.

Are there any drawbacks of Chemoprevention?

Even though many chemopreventive agents are naturally found in food, they are administered at high doses that can possibly produce unfavourable side effects. Short- and long-term side effects of chemopreventive agents are unknown at this time.

Although most chemoprevention trials show promising results, there are a few that present possible detrimental effects. One study, the Alpha-Tocopherol, Beta-Carotene Lung Cancer Prevention Study, tested daily doses of alpha-tocopherol (Vitamin E) or beta-carotene, or both, on reducing the rates of lung and other cancers in male smokers. One of the findings included a 18% increase in lung cancer in the beta-carotene group. This result stresses the importance of waiting for conclusive results and approved recommendations from the scientific world before making any lifestyle changes.

CONCLUSION

There is little evidence supporting widespread use of chemopreventive agents in the entire population. The evidence only supports risk reduction for those individuals at risk for cancer. At this time, supplements of vitamins, minerals, or other agents for the prevention of cancer have not been recommended. However, eating a well-balanced, low-fat diet including fruits, vegetables and grains has been advocated.

Chemoprevention is not simple, and successes may not come quickly. However, for individuals at high risk for cancer and possibly the general population in the future, chemoprevention has the potential of providing an important means for cancer risk reduction.

8

COMMON UROLOGICAL PROBLEMS

A.K. MANDAL* AND R.S. RAI*

It is very difficult to say that what are the most common urological problems, which really affect the healthy and happy life of an individual. In clinical urolgical practice, has been observed that problems like benign enlargement prostate, urinary stone disease; erectile dysfunction and infertility are a great concern to the individual and also take a lot time of the concerned clinician/urologist. In the ensuing article we have tried to give an account of these problems, their brief account, how to evaluate them and a guideline for the management. In case of any doubt or clarification, readers are requested to write to the author or consult a trained urologist.

Lately, we have also observed an increase in the incidence of urogenital trauma probably because of an increase in high-speed traffic and more number of automobiles on our roads. The most intriguing point is that the individual involved in these high-speed road traffic accidents are young individuals, who are in their prime of life and at times, the

*Department of Urology, PGI, Chandigarh.

sole earning member of the family. Besides having injuries to the urogenital tract, other organ system are also injured and sometimes the complete recovery of these trauma victims are not possible and they have to live with the residual deficit. Rehabilitation of these patients becomes problematic to the patient, himself, his family and as well as to the society. A collective effort is required at all levels, i.e. the individual, family, society, NGO's, the government and other law enforcing agencies to prevent and bring down the number of these accident cases.

The prostate gland is made of two parts, an inner cranial zone and outer caudal zone. Benign enlargement begins in the inner cranial zone in the collection of glands adjacent to the urethra. No man can escape the changes which begin to appear in his prostate as he grows older: by the time he is 40 years old the microscope will show scores of tiny benign foci of nodular hyperplasia scattered throughout the inner zone of the gland.

Over the next 30 years these foci gradually enlarge, coalesce and elongate the prostate, whilst compressing the prostatic urethra from side to side. The enlargement of these nodules gives rise to the so-called lobes of prostate, which are not a normal anatomical entity, but an artifact, which reflects the way the bladder neck and the shape of the bony pelvis mould the enlarging adenoma. At the same time when these changes are taking place, there is an equally important change in the smooth muscle at the neck of the bladder, which looses its normal ability to relax in coordination with the contraction of the detrusor. The result is an unyielding ring of tissue at the neck of bladder, which fails to open as the detrusor contracts. The combination of mechanical deformity and smooth muscle malfunction results in an increased resistance at the outlet of bladder.

In response to this, the detrusor muscle of the urinary bladder undergoes hypertrophy. To the naked eye the changes are obvious: the muscle thickens, and its trabeculae become coarsened and change from a fine felt work into a net through whose spaces the mucosa of the bladder is pushed out to form multiple saccules and eventually diverticula. As these changes progress further, the detrusor begins to fail. Failure may be gradual or sudden. In gradual failure, at first bladder is no longer capable of ridding itself of urine, with telltale appearance in the ultrasound and urogram of residual urine. This process may continue slowly and painlessly until one day the volume of residual urine becomes so great that the bladder begins to leak involuntarily—chronic retention with overflow. In acute failure of the detrusor the patient suddenly finds himself unable to empty the bladder. This may occur at any stage in the story, and may be precipitated by some other illness, over distention of the bladder from drunkenness or being given a diuretic.

DIAGNOSTIC APPROACH

The patients with BPH needs a well planned assessment to determine:

(i) The nature and severity of symptoms,
(ii) Whether there is objective evidence of obstruction, and
(iii) The effect of obstruction on the upper urinary tract.

A. Symptoms

Symptoms of BPH should be quantified with standardized symptom scores such as that developed by the American urological Association (AUA). The questionnaire in this scoring system consists of seven questions to quantify symptoms and sections to determine how bothersome symptoms are and assess quality of life. Although treatment should be individualized, as general rule patients with scores of 7 or less are considered to have mild symptoms that probably do not require immediate treatment unless hydronephrosis or uraemia is present. Patients with moderate symptoms (AUA scores of 8-20) probably are in need of some therapy. Patients with severe symptoms (AUA scores above 20) frequently require treatment to avoid development of complications.

B. History

A detailed urologic history should be taken assessing prior surgery, infections, strictures, stones, tumours or bleeding in the urinary tract. The general medical history should especially focus on cardiovascular disease, pulmonary disease, habits (alcohol consumption, and smoking) and about medications.

C. Physical Examination

(i) General physical examination—For general nutritional status and any telltale signs of chronic renal failure.
(ii) Abdominal examination—For any palpable flank mass or palpable bladder.
(iii) Examination of male genitalia and digital rectal examination (DRE)—The purpose of DRE is to assess prostate size, symmetry and consistency; to assess the anal tone; and to assess the presence of rectal masses.
(iv) Focused neurological examination, which should include perineal sensation and assessment of bulbocavernosus reflex.

D. Laboratory Tests

Laboratory tests should include urinalysis, urine culture, complete blood count and determination of serum creatinine, blood urea nitrogen (BUN), blood sugar and serum electrolytes for most patients. For patients with more than 50 years of age, a test for prostatic-specific antigen (PSA) is highly recommended.

E. Ultrasound

This is required to evaluate the upper tracts, assess the size and consistency of prostate and measure the volume of post-void residual urine.

F. Uroflometry

The peak flow rate is a sensitive indicator of outflow obstruction. It should always be performed in conjunction with estimation of post-void residual urine volume. The normal peak flow should be more than 12 ml/s in normal male adults voiding more than 150 ml.

TREATMENT

Regardless of the causes of BPH, it is the symptoms severity and the impact of the lower urinary tract symptoms on quality of life (QOL) that bring patient to seek urologist's attention. The goals of BPH therapy may differ based on the perspective of the individual conducting the assessment. Primary care physicians are concerned with safety of treatments used. Urologists have traditionally favoured transurethral resection of the prostate. Urodynamicists are concerned with determining whether patients have true bladder-outlet obstruction. Clinical researchers compare different treatments for efficacy and safety. Insurers and payers seek to minimize and defer treatment costs. But above all, the patient concerns should remain central in the evaluation of BPH treatment.

The classic goals of therapy for BPH are to improve symptoms, arrest the disease process and prevent some of the adverse outcomes associated with BPH, such as acute retention of urine and the need for surgery. From the patient's perspective, QOL is the major concern and symptoms improvement is the main objective. Patients prefer an oral agent to alleviate symptoms; they also favour an oral agent with minimal side effects, particularly effects that do not impair sexual function, cause impotence, or alter ejaculation. They also wish to avoid surgery and other invasive interventions; therefore, the treatment of BPH is highly individualized and depends on severity of symptoms and presence of complications in a given case. Refractory urinary retentions, upper tract deterioration, recurrent infection, haematuria and bladder stones are strong indications for intervention according to most urologists. For patients without these findings, the level of symptoms remains the main determinant of therapy and timing of intervention, if required.

1. Watchful Waiting

Watchful waiting involves careful follow-up of symptoms and signs without active intervention and is recommended for majority of patients with mild symptoms (AUA score of 0 to 7).

2. Pharmacologic Therapy

The drugs commonly used in the treatment of BPH are phenoxybenzamine, doxazosin, terazosin, alfuzosin and tamsulosin. Most of these drugs have side effects such as dizziness, lightheadedness and asthenia that are related to their antihypertensive actions except tamsulosin. From 50% to 75% of patient experience rapid improvement in symptoms with pharmalogic therapy.

3. Phytotherapy

Phytotherapy consists of administration of plant extracts; the mechanism of most of these extracts is not fully understood. The commonly used extracts are from saw palmetto, *Pygeum africanum*, South African star grass, root of *Hypoxis rooperi*, fruits of *Sebal serulata*, leaves of trembling poplar, fruits of *Cucubita pepo*, roots of *Echinacea purpurea*, etc.

4. Trans Urethral Prostectomy (TURP)

This remains one of the most effective treatments for BPH. The prostate is resected by electrocautery from within the prostatic urethra. The common complications associated with this procedure are urethral strictures (10%), bladder neck contracture (10%), epididymitis or orchitis (2%), permanent incontinence (1%) and erectile impotence (5%). Retrograde ejaculation occurs in approximately 50% of patients and should be discussed fully with the patient during the process of obtaining informed consent.

5. Laser Prostectomy

It offers several advantages over TURP including lower morbidity and mortality rates, cost savings and can be performed on the out-patient basis. This procedure is also performed transurethrally, the most commonly used laser is Ho: YAG laser. The entire adenomatous zone is enucleated into the bladder and subsequently the adenoma is morcellated out from the bladder.

6. Open Prostectomy

As in TURP, only the hyperplasic adenoma and not the entire prostate is removed. The common indications for open prostectomy are prostatic enlargement more than 60 G, presence of bladder calculi not amenable to transurethral lithotripsy and presence of bladder diverticula requiring excision. The choice of operative approach depends on the surgeon's preference, although there are other considerations that apply.

7. Other Less Common Procedure

(a) Transurethral incision of prostate (TUIP).
(b) Transurethral vaporization of prostate (TUVP).
(c) Intraprostatic stents.
(d) Balloon dilatation of prostate (BDP).
(e) Transurethral microwave therapy (TUMT).
(f) Transurethral needle ablation (TUNA).
(g) High intensity focused ultrasound (HIFU).

URINARY STONES

The occurrence of stones within the urinary tract is a problem that has plagued humans since the beginning of recorded history. Archaeologists have uncovered urinary stones in the mummified remains of Egyptians estimated to be more than 7,000 years old. The exact incidence of stone disease is not exactly known in India; its incidence differs from one region to the other. In the USA, stone disease accounts for more than 4,000,000 hospital admissions annually. The peak incidence is in the third to fifth decades. Men are affected three times as commonly as women. In a patient who has passed one stone, the likelihood of passing another stone is about 15% by 3 years and 30% by 15 years. Formation of stone (Urolithiasis) is a life long problem, with an average of 9 years intervening between episodes. The various factors associated with urolithiasis are enumerated in Table 1.

Causes of Stone Formation

Stone formation is heterogeneous disorder with varying chemical composition and pathophysiological background. Although stones are generally composed of calcium oxalate or calcium phosphate, they may also consist of uric acid,

Table I

Factors Associated with Urolithiasis

Factor	*Conditions of increased incidence*
Genetics/heredity	Cystinuria-autosomal recessive
	Renal tubular acidosis-type I
	Medullary sponge kidney
Geography	High temperature/humidity
Diet	Increased intake of calcium or oxalate
Occupation	Sedentary jobs

magnesium-ammonium phosphate or cystine. Stones develop from a wide variety of metabolic or environmental disturbances, including various forms of hypercalciurias, hypocitraturia, undue urinary acidity, hyperuricosuria, hyperoxaluria, infection with urease-producing organism and cystinuria. The cause of stone formation may be determined in most patients using the reliable diagnostic protocols that are available for identification of these disturbances.

Clinical Presentation

Kidney stones are usually silent until the stone moves within the urinary tract and produces either blood (haematuria) or some degree of urinary obstruction. This may be accompanied by pain, urinary infection generalized sepsis, nausea or vomiting. Pain may radiate to the groin, testes, or tip of the penis, depending upon the location of obstruction. In 25% of cases, patients give a family story of stone disease.

Diagnosis

Initial evaluation includes urinalysis, urine culture and plain X-ray of abdomen (KUB). More than two-thirds of urinary calculi are radiopaque and can be seen on the X-ray. The initial radiologic investigation should be a renal ultrasound (US). This may demonstrate the presence of stone as well as any evidence of hydronephrosis. An axial or spiral computerized tomography (CT) will confirm the presence of calculus in the urinary tract and demonstrate the degree of obstruction. The spiral CT is rapid, does not require a bowel preparation, and avoids the use of intravenous contrast. It is very accurate at identifying stones in the collecting system and ureter.

Treatment

The diagnosis and management of urolithiasis has undergone considerable evolution in recent years. About 90% of stones that cause renal colic pass spontaneously. All patients with stone disease should be advised to increased fluid intake, limit dietary protein and limit sodium. The initial management is based on three key concepts:

1. The recognition of urgent and emergency requirements for urologic consultations.
2. The provision of effective pain control using a combination of narcotics and non-steroidal anti-inflammatory drugs in appropriate patients.
3. An understanding of the impact of stone location and size on natural history and definitive urologic management.

For proper therapy of stone disease it is extremely important to determine stone characteristics such as type, size, location, and underlying metabolic abnormalities as therapy is often dependent on these features. Treatment of acute episode depends on the size and location of the stone, degree of obstruction and patient clinical status.

1. Indication for Intervention

Patients with infection or high-grade obstruction require prompt intervention. This usually requires passage of retrograde ureteral catheter or percutaneous nephrostomy drainage. Patients with small stones and minimal hydronephrosis may be treated conservatively as out-patients with oral hydration and analgesics. About 90% of ureteric calculi measuring less than 4 mm in diameter pass spontaneously, whereas only 20% of stone greater than 6 mm in diameter pass.

2. Expectant Treatment

It is indicated in the asymptomatic, non-obstructed, non-infected patient with a stone less than 4 mm in diameter in the lower third of urine. Four to six weeks should be allowed for stone passage.

3. Stone Extraction

It is indicated for lower ureteral stones that do not pass spontaneously. Most of these stones can be extracted endoscopically. Several options are available. Small stones may be grasped directly or engaged in a stone basket and extracted. Larger stones may be fragmented using US, electohydraulic, pneumatic or a laser lithotripsy. Success rates are approximately 90%.

4. Shock Wave lithotripsy (SWL)

Although its primary use is in the fragmentation of renal calculi, SWL is also advantageous for ureteral stones, especially those less than 8 mm in diameter. SWL may be performed either with or without a stent in place, as long as the stone can be adequately visualized.

5. Ureterolithotomy

It is rarely necessary, given the high success rate of non-operative and minimally invasive techniques, such as SWL, ureteroscopy and laparascopy.

6. Percutaneous Nephrolithtomy (PCNL)

In this procedure, an antegrade puncture is made into the pelvicalyceal system of kidney under image intensifier after outlining the system by contrast media. The ensuing tract is dilated and stones are removed after fragmenting it either by a lithoclast, ultrasonic lithotriptor or laser. The remaining residual significant fragments, which are inaccessible, can further be subjected to ESWL fragmentation and spontaneous clearance.

7. Surgery

Most of the renal or ureteral stones can be removed by ESWL/PCNL or by a combination of both. However, in certain situation like large stone bulk, poorly functioning stone, any associated anatomic abnormality, conventional open surgery still has a role.

BLADDER STONES

Bladder stones are most often found in male patients and are caused by bladder outlet obstruction are foreign bodies (portions of catheters, sutures, or objects inserted through the urethra). Ureteral stones that reach the bladder can also act as a nidus for bladder stone formation. Bladder stones are composed of variable proportions of calcium oxalate, uric acid and ammonium urate. If the uric acid ids a major component, bladder stones may be radiolucent. They vary from extremely hard to quite soft. Patients with long standing bladder stones are at risk for squamous metaplasia or carcinoma.

Clinical presentation includes pain felt in the lower part of abdomen or referred to penis, intermittent stream, dysuria and haematuria. Patients may also present with recurrent urinary tract infections.

Diagnosis includes plain film of the abdomen and US of bladder. Cystoscopy is usually performed in conjunction with treatment.

Treatment

1. Lithotrites

Lithotrites are mechanical devices that permit crushing of large, hard bladder stones under direct vision. The fragments are then washed out through a resectoscope sheath.

2. Electrohydraulic Lithotripsy

It is based on the principle of underwater spark generation. The lithotripsy probe produces a hydraulic shock wave near the stone that usually produces fragmentation after delivery of several shocks.

3. US Lithotripsy

It is based on US energy delivered through a rigid probe

passed through an endoscope. Small fragments are removed by continuous suction attached to the hollow US probe.

4. Cystolithotomy

It can be performed through a small suprapubic incision. It has the advantage of removing the entire stone rather than leaving the fragments in the bladder.

5. Percutaneous Cystolithotomy (PCCL)

In this procedure a percutaneous puncture is made in the bladder, the tract is dilated and stone is removed after fragmentation.

ERECTILE DYSFUNCTION (ED) IN MALE

Erectile dysfunction or sexual dysfunction in male is defined as the persistent inability to obtain and maintain an erection sufficient for sexual intercourse. It is more prevalent among patients with atherosclerotic peripheral vascular disease, hypertension, diabetes mellitus, hypercholesterolemia and heart disease and among men who smoke cigarettes.

Sexual function serves deeply felt personal needs, reinforces the permanence of pair-bonding in couples, and aids in the stability of society in general, in addition, if this is deranged, the sexual dysfunction may cause substantial emotional concerns in the patient but most patients hesitate to seek medical intervention with complaints of sexual dysfunction. In addition, when finally medical intervention is sought, the patient may be discussing the physician a subject that he can not discuss even with his closest friends or sexual partner. Sexual function is a complex behaviour involving 4 integrated sequential stages desire, arousal, orgasm and resolution in which each compotent is neither singly necessary nor sufficient. Disturbance in any phase can be primary, secondary, and tertiary or halo effect either singly or in combination. Men affected with sexual dysfunction are depressed or anxious about having such a problem and may resort to going to bed late, drinking excessively or starting an argument with their partner in order to avoid a sexual encounter. Relationship difficulties may surface affecting the sexual activity of the person. The couple may begin to avoid contact and drift apart because of isolation or frustration. Loss of self-esteem may extend into their job performances and interactions with others. Epidemiological studies report a 30 to 40% prevalence of sexual dysfunction in the general population, which varies by phase of sexual dysfunction, gender, age, education, health, lifestyle, relationship status, etc.

Primary impotence refers to impotence that is life-long, whereas **secondary** impotence implies the loss of previously normal potency. Impotence caused exclusively by emotional stress or psychiatric disease is termed **psychiatric** impotence and accounts for an estimates 10% to 50% of all impotence. **Organic** impotence, which is erectile dysfunction caused exclusively by vascular, neurologic, endocrine or other physical diseases accounts for an estimated 50% to 80% of cases. In majority of impotent men, erectile impairment has both a psychological and an organic basis and a complete management program is required.

Etiology of Impotence

The causes of impotence are summarized as given below:

I. Psychogenic
II. Organic

(a) *Inflammatory*: prostatitis, urethritis, stricture.
(b) *Mechanical*: chordee, Peyronie's disease, phimosis.
(c) *Postoperative*: iatrogenic, aortic or peripheral vascular surgery, renal transplantation, pelvic irradiation, abdomonioperineal resection of rectum, transurethral sphincterotomy, cavernosal-spongiosal shunts, radical prostectomy or cystoprostectomy, neurosurgical procedures like lumbar laminectomy, sacral rhizotomy and pudendal neurectomy.
(d) *Occlusive:* Arteriogenic—atherosclerosis: The general vascular risk factors include hypertension, cigarette smoking, diabetes mellitus and hypercholesterolemia.

Venogenic: results from fibrosis of the erectile tissues resulting in decreased expandability with subsequent poor stretching of the subtunical venules, poor venous outflow resistance and failure to maintain erection. Ischemia may be secondary to atherosclerosis, pelvic or perineal injuries or injuries to the penis that occur while the penis is erect (fractured penis).

(e) *Traumatic*: pelvic fracture, urethral rupture, perineal trauma.

(f) *Endurance*: chronic and systemic disease, e.g. chronic renal failure.

(g) *Neurologic*: neuropathy, Parkinson's disease, cerebrovascular accidents, temporal lobe epilepsy, multiple sclerosis, spinal cord trauma, myelodysplasia.

(h) *Chemical*: alcohol, marijuana, prescription drugs.

(i) *Endocrine*: diabetes mellitus, testicular failure, pituitary failure, hyperprolactenemia.

Evaluation

This includes:

A. Sexual History

The onset, duration and circumstances of the erection problem are all important. One can distinguish three different types of erections: partner-induced, nocturnal and self-induced (masturbation). The three important qualities of erection are hardness, maintenance and spontaneity. It is useful to ask the patient questions concerning the qualities of all three types of erection.

B. Detailed Medical History.

C. Psychological Evaluation

A psychological interview with a psychologist or sex therapist is used to assess the presence of personality disorder and anxiety. If possible, the couple should be present for the evaluation to assess their expectations from the planned therapy.

D. Physical Examination

The general body habitus and status of secondary sexual characteristics should be assessed. Gynaecomastia may be present in patients with androgen deficiency or estrogen excess. The penis should be examined carefully for adequacy of length, fibrotic regions of the tunica albuginea or deformities of corporal bodies.

E. Laboratory Tests

Laboratory tests should routinely include a complete blood count, determination of blood sugar, serum creatinine and liver function tests. Hormonal status is adequately assessed by serum testosterone, luteinizing hormone and serum prolactin levels. If both luteinizing hormone and testosterone levels are decreased, hypogonadotrophic hypogonadism is suspected and warrants consultation with endocrinologist.

F. Specialized Tests

- ❑ Nocturnal penile tumescence test (NPT) refers to the assessment of changes in penile circumference that occur during sleep. Such testing may be done to distinguish organic from psychogenic impotence, but its validity remains controversial. Overall, the accuracy of NPT in distinguishing organic from psychogenic impotence is approximately 80%. Formal NPT testing is usually performed in a sleep laboratory and is thus somewhat impractical and costly.
- ❑ Neurologic testing. Penile boithesiometry is used to assess the threshold for vibratory sensation. This is a very limited test because it is not neurophysiologic.
- ❑ Vascular testing. This includes:
  - (i) Penile-brachial index testing.
  - (ii) Duplex ultrasonography.
  - (iii) Dynamic infusion cavernosometry and cavernosography.
  - (iv) Selective internal pudendal arteriography.

Treatment

A. Sex Therapy

Patients with evidence of psychogenic impotence and not discernible organic cause should be encouraged to undergo a short course (6 to 12 weeks) of sex therapy.

B. Non-surgical Therapy

1. The vacuum erection device (VED) is considered one of the three main forms of therapy for ED. The VED is best suited to the patient who wants non-invasive treatment. The advantage of VED includes simplicity of use, low cost, relative safety, and ability to start treatment immediately.

2. Intracavernous pharmacotherapy. Most patients suffering from ED, both organic and mixed may potentially be treated intracavernous pharmacotherapy. The commonly used drug is alprostadyl, which can be taken alone or in combination with papaverine and/or phentolamine mesylate. Most studies show increased efficacy for the three-drug combination regime compared with monotherapy. Patients are usually advised to inject a maximal of three times per week.

3. Transurethral alprostadyl (Medicated urethral system for erection—MUSE). A medicated pellet containing alprostadyl is inserted intraurethrally with an applicator. Recent studies suggest that application of a ring may enhance intracavernosal drug delivery.

4. Oral drugs.

- Sildanefil citrate-acts by inhibiting the cGMP specific phosphodiesterase type V. The result is an increase in intracellular concentration of cGMP and amplification of corporal smooth muscle relaxation.
- Phentolamine
- Apomorphine
- Androgen replacement-indicated only in-patient with documented androgen deficiency.

C. Surgical Therapy

Vascular Surgery

Patients with "failure-to-fill" erectile dysfunction and focal arteriogenic pathology are candidates for penile revascularization. Most ideal candidates are young men with a history of perineal or pelvic trauma in whom arteriography reveals a localized common penile artery problem. Revascularization is achieved by microsurgical anastomosis of the inferior epigastric artery to the dorsal penile artery.

Inflatable Prostheses

Excellent functional and cosmetic results can be achieved with multicomponent penile prostheses. Inflatable prostheses consist of a pair of inflatable cylinders, a reservoir, a pump, and tubing to connect these components. Compressing the pumps achieves active transfer of fluid from the reservoir into the cylinders. Pressing a release valve on the pump allows passive flow of fluid back to the reservoir and achieves detumescence.

Non-inflatable Prostheses

In general, these devices do not provide the cosmetic results achieved by the multicomponent inflatable devices, but the lower cost and relative ease of insertion make them desirable in selected cases.

MALE INFERTILITY

Infertility is defined as the inability to achieve a pregnancy resulting in live birth after 1 year of unprotected intercourse (primary infertility). Couples by whom fewer than desired numbers of children are produced have secondary infertility. Approximately 15% of couples cannot achieve an unassisted pregnancy. A male factor can be identified in nearly 50% of these couples (one-third male factor only and 20% joint subfertility).

Evaluation of the Infertile Couple

It has been observed that while treating infertile couples,

the physician generally deals with young, healthy persons who are nevertheless faced with a profound organic dysfunction: inability to procreate. The best approach is direct, factual, and sensitive to the psychological implications of infertility.

A. History

Information regarding the duration of marriage and attempts to conceive is essential in establishing that infertility exists. If either partner has been previously married, it is important to determine whether one or more pregnancies resulted, and if not, what the reasons were. A survey of the sexual development of the male partner during childhood and puberty, including information about undescended testicles, hypospadias, gynaecomastia, mumps, herniorraphy, scrotal surgery and the onset of pubertal changes are important. A history of retrograde ejaculation usually caused in diabetic autonomic neuropathy, sympatholytic drugs or retroperitoneal surgery is equally important. A history of urethritis or epididymitis may suggest genital tract obstruction as cause for infertility. Cigarette smoking has adverse effects on the sperm count, motility and morphology. The spermatogenic function of the testis is extremely sensitive to radiation and may be completely destroyed by as little as 80 cGy. Sometimes self-administered drugs may be detrimental to the process of spermatogenesis, especially marijuana and alcohol.

B. Physical Examination

Physical examination in an infertile male patient may provide a specific diagnosis or suggest the focus for the ensuing workup. The examination is best performed with the patient standing in a warm room.

- ❑ Testes—the size and consistency.
- ❑ Spermatic cord—any asymmetry should be noted. The presence of both vasa must be clearly documented. Bilateral absence of both vasa is rare but may occur in up to 2% of infertile male patients. Both spermatic cords should be palpated for the presence of varicoceles.

- Abnormalities of the urethral meatus or any penile anatomic features that could interfere with normal intercourse and delivery of ejaculation to the vagina should be evaluated.
- It is also important to examine the body habitus and the presence of gynaecomastia or galactorrhea (possible indicators of excess circulating estrogens) must be noted.

C. Laboratory Evaluation

- Semen analysis is the single most important component of the Laboratory evaluation of the infertile male patient. The semen should be collected after 3 days of abstinence from ejaculation; the specimen should be kept at room temperature and delivered to the laboratory within 1 hour.
- Fructose assay—an absence of fructose in the azoospermic patient indicates either bilateral seminal vesicle aplasia or bilateral ejaculatory duct obstruction.
- Sperm density, morphology and function.
- Testicular biopsy.

Other tests, which may be required to analyze sperm function, are:

- *In vitro* mucus penetration tests.
- *In vivo* penetration tests.
- *In vitro* fertilization testing.
- Sperm antibody tests.

Hormonal Assays

- Follicular stimulating hormone (FSH), luteinizing hormone (LH) and testosterone are routinely measured to detect abnormalities in the hypothalamic-pituitary-testicular axis, which account for a small percentage of patients with infertility.

- Prolactin. An elevated level of prolactin secondary to a pituitary microadenoma may result in suppression of FSH and LH output and is usually suspected when symptoms and signs of testosterone deficiency are noted.

Enumerating the various treatment options depending upon the causes of infertility in a given case is beyond the scope of this article. Treatment of an infertile male/couple involves highly specialized techniques ranging from ligation of varicoceles, correction of obstructive azoospermia (vaso-vasostomy, vaso-epididymal anastomosis) to procedures like *in vitro* fertilization-embryo transfer (IVF-ET), intacytoplasmic sperm injection (ICSI) employed in artificial reproduction. With these procedures a pregnancy rate of 40-47% can be achieved in the infertile couples.

9

HEALTHY LIFESTYLE AND PREVENTION OF DISEASES OF JOINTS AND BONES

RAJ BAHADUR*

I. INTRODUCTION

As we grow in age, the bony tissues and the joints where they meet tend to lose some of their hardness and smoothness respectively. With the result the bones become soft and porous. Such bones can break more easily with the loss of smoothness inside the joints, the capacity to move the joint is compromised and/or the movements become painful and restricted. The former condition is called osteoporosis (bone softening) and the latter is called osteoarthritis (joint degeneration). However, this deterioration with age is neither consistent nor inevitable. Age is not the only factor, to determine the fate of bones and joints. Several faulty lifestyle factors can lead to exceleration of loss and healthy lifestyle.

* Professor and Head, Department of Orthopedics, GMC&H, Sector 32, Chandigarh.

2. MUSCULO-SKELETAL PROBLEMS ASSOCIATED WITH SEDANTARY LIFESTYLE AND AGEING

Ageing is a progressive loss of adaptation as time passes. Elderly people are less able to adapt and need more help in recovering from disease and injury than younger counterparts. Elderly population is considered to be 65 years of age and older. The increase in life expectancy has lead to increase in the population of ageing population and their associated problems including rise in health care costs. Though ageing and faulty lifestyle affect the entire body, a brief discussion about musckoskeletal effects, i.e. osteoarthritis and osteoporosis shall be discussed. The other common musculo-skeletal problems in the elderly include degenerated disease of the spine leading to lumbar and cervical spondylosis. Old age may reduce activity, but it is the mental attitude to exercise, which is important.

3. OSTEOARTHRITIS

There is a consistently documented association of inactive lifestyle and ageing and primary osteoarthritis. Clinically, the disease presents as joint pains without systemic effects. Osteoarthritis can be classified into primary (idiopathic) and secondary osteoarthritis. In idiopathic osteoarthritis, there is no predisposing factor whereas there is an obvious underlying cause in secondary osteoarthritis like prior injury to the joint. Primary osteoarthritis is the most common joint disease of human beings and a leading cause of disability in the elderly. The Common Sites of Idiopathic (Primary) Osteoarthritis include knee, hands and spine. However, regular and proper exercises can keep the muscles and the underlying joints in a good health and prevent their deterioration.

3.1 Pathophysiology

Pathologically the disease processes not only affect the articular cartilage which is the glistening surface of joint providing frictionless movements at joint, but also involves the other joint structures. The disease is characterized by irregular wearing out of cartilage, more in the areas of increased load and also by changes in adjacent subchondral bone and synovial inflammation (swelling of the joint). Later there is total loss of cartilage.

Muscle spasm, joint instability leading to capsular stretching, micro-fractures and synovitis may be the cause of pain.

3.2 Risk Factors for Osteoarthritis

Besides laziness, old age, female sex, major joint trauma, obesity, congenital or developmental defects, are considered to be risk factors in development of osteoarthritis.

Racial differences are seen in the prevalence of osteoarthritis and the pattern of joint involvement. It has been seen that Chinese and Indians have a lower incidence of osteoarthritis of hip and more incidence of knee osteoarthritis as compared to the Whites. Whether these differences are genetic or relate to cultural differences in joint usage is not clear.

3.3 Clinical Features

Osteoarthritis usually affects a single joint or only a few joints in contrast to rheumatoid arthritis, which tends to involve multiple joints. Joints pain usually the first symptom and leads the patient to seek medical advice, which is often described as cheep ache, localized to the joint. Typically, the pain is aggravated by use and relieved by test but as the disease progresses, even rest pain may appear. Morning stiffness of the involved joint usually lasts less than 20 minutes as compared to rheumatoid arthritis where it lasts more than 30 minutes.

3.4 Osteoarthritis at Specific Joint Sites

3.4.1 Interphalangeal Joints

Heberden's nodes, bony enlargements of the distal interphalangeal joints, are amongst the most common presentation of idiopathic osteoarthritis. These nodes develop gradually, with little or no discomfort in earlier stages, however, they may present acutely with pain, redness and swelling sometimes triggered by minor trauma. Joint deformity and functional impairment may be severe in late stages.

3.4.2 Thumb Base

Carpo-metacarpal joint (trapezio-metacarpal) at the base of the thumb is a frequently involved site. Thumb base osteoarthritis may cause loss of motion and strength, pain on pinching motion. It also leads to deformity of the thumb, a swan neck deformity.

3.4.3 The Knee

Knee is the single most commonly affected joint by idiopathic osteoarthritis in Indian elderly population. Squatting and sitting cross legged as is prevalent in the Indian culture is thought to increase the stress across the knee joint and is a contributing factor in development of primary osteoarthritis of the knee. Osteoarthritis affecting the knee may lead to bow leg deformity. Obesity and decreasing walking habits appear to contribute a great deal.

3.4.4 The Spine

Degenerative disease of the spine can involve the facets of joints and intervertebral discs. Symptoms of spinal osteoarthritis include localized pain and stiffness and radicular pain due to nerve root compression by an osteophyte blocking a neural foramen.

3.4.5 Generalized Osteoarthritis

Generalized osteoarthritis is characterized by involvement of three or more joints or group of joints. The erythrocyte sedimentation rate may be elevated, but serum rheumatoid factor tests are negative which helps to differentiate if from rheumatoid arthritis.

3.4.6 Radiographic Features

The First radiological finding is usually joint space narrowing. Other radiographic findings include marginal osteophytes which are hotly outgrowths. Subluxation or dislocation may be seen in advanced disease.

Approaches such as magnetic resonance imaging (MRI) and ultrasonography are expensive and are not necessary.

3.5 Treatment

Treatment is aimed at reducing pain, maintaining mobility, and minimizing disability. Treatment of osteoarthritis should be individualized and tailored to the severity of symptoms and the requirements of the patient. In individuals with mild symptoms, treatment may be limited to patient education, physical and occupational therapy and topical analgesics. In more severe involvement, the use of analgesics may be added. Judicious use of intra-articular injections also has a role. Patients with severe symptomatic osteoarthritis require an aggressive, generally surgical approach.

The treatment modalities may be broadly classified into:

- Non-pharmacological therapy
- Pharmacological therapy
- Systemic
- Local
- Surgery

3.6 Non-pharmacological Therapy

3.6.1 Exercise

The aim is to reduce impairment and improve function. This can be often achieved by muscle strengthening exercises, which helps to achieve a better control of the muscles over a particular joint. Thus, it has been seen that patients of osteoarthritis of the knee greatly benefit from Quadriceps strengthening exercises, which helps to reduce stress on the paello-femoral joint.

In addition mobilization exercises help to maintain the mobility of the joint. These exercises have a great role in prevention and management of osteoarthritis.

3.6.2 Weight Loss

Weight reduction in patients who are obese often results in reduction of pain and improvement in function of weight hearing joints; as well as decreased requirement of analgesics.

3.6.3 Physical Modalities

Applications of local heat have been widely employed or pain relief in osteoarthritis.

3.6.4 Orthotic Devices

Wedged insoles may be useful in management of osteoarthritis of the knees. These reduce excessive loading on the medial compartment of the knee and strain on the lateral collateral ligament. Use of a stick in the opposite hand helps to reduce the loading on the affected hip.

3.6.5 Patient Education and Ergonomic Care

For effective management, encouragement, reassurance, advice about exercise, and recommendation of measures to unload the arthritic joint may be all that is required. Patients with osteoarthritis of the knee should avoid kneeling and squatting. Rest periods during day may be at benefit but complete immobilization of the painful joint is rarely indicated.

3.6.6 Pharmacological Therapy for Osteoarthritis Pain

In management of osteoarthritis pain, pharmacological agents should be used as adjuncts to non-pharmacological measures.

Analgesic Therapy

(i) Non-specific NSAIDS

Non-steroidal anti-inflammatory drugs are analgesic and anti-inflammatory with their predominant mechanism of action by the inhibition of prostaglandin biosynthesis. Commonly used drugs include Ibuprofen, diclofenac, piroxicam, indoivinethacin, aspirin, etc.

(ii) Specific COX-2 Inhibitor NSAIDs (Analgesics)

Inhibition of prostaglandin synthesis by non-specific NSAIDs also leads to inhibition of the enzyme, cyclo-oxygenase-I (COX-I), which is responsible also for adverse effects of these drugs like GI adverse effects. Selective COX-2 specific inhibitors like meloxicam, celecoxib, rofecoxib and valdecoxib are available and have better GI tolerance.

(iii) Opioids

They deserve consideration for acute flares of joint pain when an NSAIDs do not produce adequate analgesia, however their long-term use can cause drug dependence.

3.6.7 Local Therapy

(i) Rubefacients

Application of topical counter-irritants to the painful joint and muscles and the local heat provided by rubefacients may be beneficial.

(ii) Intra-articular Injection of Corticosteroid

It is a reasonable choice in patients with osteoarthritis, especially in non-weight bearing joints. Although, clinical experience with intra-articular steroid therapy supports its safety, rapidly progressive joint degeneration has been observed after frequent, repeated injunctions in large doses into the same joint.

(ii) Intra-articular Injection of Hyaluronic Acid

lntra-articular injections of hyaluronic acid are a recent introduction. In osteoarthritis, the concentration and molecular weight (MW) of synovial fluid hyaluronic acid are reduced and the viscoelastic properties of the fluid compromised. Injections of exogenous hyaluronic acid into the joint appears to restore the visco-elasticity of the synovial fluid, thins giving adequate joint lubrication.

3.6.8 Disease Modifying Drugs for Osteoarthritis

Drugs that may prevent or retard the progression of articular cartilage breakdown in osteoarthritis are now receiving increasing attention. Such agents have been called "chondroprotective" drugs. Glueosamine amid chondroitin sulfate are two such agents available. Both these agents cause synthesis of new cartilage and repair the damaged cartilage. They also protect existing cartilage from premature breakdown by inhibiting the action of certain cartilage destroying enzymes.

3.6.9 Surgery

Surgical option should be reserved for patients with advanced osteoarthritis in whom aggressive medical management has failed. Although a variety of surgical procedures, e.g. osteotomy (bony operation to correct deformity) and arthrodesis (joint fusion) may be helpful in individual cases, overwhelmingly, surgical intervention for osteoarthritis means total joint arthroplasty, especially for the major lower limb joints. Total hip and knee arthroplasties, and arthroplasties of fingers are highly successful.

It should also be noted that a number of investigative surgical procedures, such as use of mesenchymal stem cells, and autologous osteochondral plugs (mosaicplasty) are being evaluated. None of these procedures, however, is currently indicated for treatment of osteoarthritis.

4. OSTEOPOROSIS

Osteoporosis is defined as decrease in the mass of mineralized bone per unit volume of bone, i.e. decreased density of bone.

In order to understand the osteoporosis, the structure of bone should be understood first. The bone consists of 30% organic and 70% inorganic material. The inorganic material further consists mainly of calcium and phosphate. The organic components consists mainly of collagen. In osteoporosis, both the collagen content as well as the mineral content decrease whereas in osteomalacia, only the mineral content decreases. Bony tissue in the body could be cancellous bone found at the ends of long bones (trabacular) or cortical (compact) bone, found at the shafts of long bones.

4.1 Pathophysiology

The bone is living tissue and undergoes remodeling throughout the life of an individual. The bone is formed by the osteoblasts (bone forming cells) and is continuously being resorbed by the osteoclasts (bone resorbing cells). During life time two processes continue side by side and there is a balance between the two. Peak bone mass is attained by 35 years of age after which the bone mass starts decreasing.

The factors which help to increase the bone mass include physical activity, somatostatin (growth hormone), sex hormones (estrogen, progesterone and androgens), cacitonin, Vitamin D and calcium. It is worthwhile to mention here that people who are engaged in heavy physical activities rarely suffer from osteoporosis. The factors that cause negative bone balance include parathomone, corticosteroids, and hyperthyroidism and act by stimulating osteoclastic resorption of bone and of course lack of regular exercises.

The osteoporosis can be primary or involutional, which is age related, or secondary, which is secondary to some cause like steroid intake and asthma, etc. the involutional osteoporosis, which affects the elderly can be further sub-classified into two.

4.2 Type I Osteoporosis

In type I osteoporosis, also known as post-menopausal osteoporosis, there is increased osteoelastic activity leading to more bone resorption than can be formed. The osteoblastic activity remains normal. This type of osteoporosis involves the cancellous bone amid affects as the name suggests, post-menopausal females, generally within 5 years after menopause; however, it can also affect males in the ratio of 1:6. It affects mainly cancellous bone.

4.2 Type II Osteoporosis

In type II osteoporosis, also known as senile osteoporosis, there is decreased osteoblastic activity. The osteoclastic activity remains normal. It affects both men and women in the ratio of 1:2. It affects both cortical and cancellous bone. Elderly of more than 70 years of age are generally affected by this form of osteoporosis.

4.4 Clinical Features

Osteoporosis is a silent killer with few symptoms till it causes complications, which are in the form of fractures resulting from minor trauma. Occasionally it may present with generalized bony pains. Patients with senile osteoporosis trinity present with hump back and/or decrease in height because of collapse of multiple vertebrae. The common presentations of type I osteoporosis includes vertebral fractures, distal radius fractures, peri-alveolar bone loss leading to tooth loss. The common presentations of type II osteoporosis include vertebral fractures, hip fractures, proximal tibial and proximal humerus fractures.

4.5 Diagnosis

The diagnosis of osteoporosis is essentially radiological. However, a strong clinical suspicion should be kept in the elderly. The following investigations can be done to establish the diagnosis of osteoporosis:

1. Plain X-rays

It can give idea about, osteoporosis, but it is generally difficult to quantify the extent of osteoporosis. It may reveal decreased density and pencil lining of cortex. However, the specific X-ray investigations, which are generally done, are the Singh's index (X-ray pelvis with both hips), vertebral index and calcaneal index. Plain radiographs are usually the first investigation on which osteoporosis is discovered as a co-incidental finding.

2. Bone Densitometry Measurements

It provide accurate means of assessing the osteoporosis. The bone mass is calculated using standardized scoring system according to the criteria given by WHO. In this, the calculation is done by comparing the bone density of the individual with that of standard reference young adult population and thus 'T' score is calculated. A 'T' score of less than –2.5 indicates osteoporosis whereas that between –1 to –2.5 indicates osteopenia. Bone densitometry can be done by following methods:

(a) X-ray Absorptiometry

It can be single energy or dual energy absorptiometry (DEXA), the dual energy being more accurate.

(b) Quantitative CT

It can be single energy or dual energy. It is one of the most accurate non-invasive methods to measure bone density.

(c) Quantitative Ultrasound

It is one of the most popular and inexpensive method used for screening of population for osteoporosis.

3. *Histology*

Histology is a reliable but invasive method.

4. *Biochemical Markers*

Biochemical markers for bone resorption like urinary deoxy-pyrodinoline are useful for differentiating type I from type II osteoporosis.

4.6 Management

Management includes musculoskeletal rehabilitation, various drugs and treatment of complications.

4.6.1 Musculoskeletal Rehabilitation

Musculoskeletal rehabilitation includes maintenance of skeletal mass and integrity. Skeletal loading exercises and continued physical activity help in both prevention and treatment of osteoporosis. Management of an established case includes muscle strengthening exercises and assistive devices like walking stick to minimize the chances of fall thus preventing fractures.

4.6.2 Pharmacological Approaches

Various pharmacological agents include estrogens, bisphosphonates, calcitonin, fluorides, anabolic steroids, calcium and Vitamin D.

(i) Estrogens

Estrogens cause inhibition of osteoclasts and are thus useful in type I osteoporosis in females. Administration can be in form of oral medication on skin patches. Estrogens can cause withdrawal bleeding and should be combined with progesterone. Rahoxifene, which has selective estrogen like action on the bone is a recent introduction and does not cause withdrawal uterine bleeding.

(ii) Bisphosphonates

Bisphosphonates cause inhibition of osteoclasts and are useful in type I osteoporosis. The drug needs to be given empty stomach for its absorption and may cause oesophiagitis. Alendronate is one such drug, which is commonly used.

(iii) Calcitonin

Calcitonin causes inhibition of osteoclasts and thus is useful in type I osteoporosis. It is administered as injections or as nasal spary. Calcitonin has excellent activity against bone pains associated with osteoporosis.

(iv) Anabolic Steroids

Their role in osteoporosis is empirical. They may have a role in both types I and II osteoporosis. Administration is in form of injections (nandrolone) or oral route (stanozolol). Anabolic steroids may cause liven toxicity.

(v) Fluorides

They render the bone less susceptible to osteoclastic resorption. Fluoride has a role in both types I and II osteoporosis. However, excess intake of fluoride may lead to fluorosis. Moreover the bone thus formed is more hand but brittle also.

(vi) Calcium and Vitamin D

Calcium and Vitamin D are used as adjuncts to other anti-osteoporotic drugs. Vitamin D may have some role in senile osteoporosis where its absorption is impaired more so in the elderly.

5. FRACTURE MANAGEMENT

Details of fracture management are beyond the scope of this article. Most common fractures associated with osteoporosis are vertebral, hip and distal radius fractures. Vertebral fractures are generally not associated with any neural deficit and are treated by rest for short periods, heat, analgesics followed by mobilization. Wrist fractures require POP casting after closed reduction whereas hip fractures are treated by surgical means.

6. PREVENTION

With an active and healthy lifestyle one can prevent the twin problems of osteoarthritis and osteoporosis. The exercise should be undertaken religiously. Intake of calcium and Vitamin D is essential for the health of bones and joints. Don't put on weight. Avoid smoking, alcohol, colas, coffiene, drugs, etc. Consult your physician for better health of bones, during childhood, at menopause and when the ageing sets in.

10

HEALTHY LIFESTYLE AND PREVENTION OF DISEASES OF EAR, NOSE AND THROAT

A.K. GUPTA* AND N. MATHUR

The predominant way of life in society is central to health promotion, since it fosters personal behaviour patterns that are either beneficial or detrimental to health. The promotion of lifestylès conductive to health involves consideration of personal coping strategies and dispositions as well as beliefs and values relevant to health, all shaped by lifelong experiences and living conditions.

Many of the diseases affecting the ears, nose and throat in an individual are linked with the person's lifestyle. These diseases can be either prevented or their effects can be diminished by improving the living conditions of the individual.

Good personal hygiene is a essence of health body. People especially children having poor body hygiene and those living in unhygienic surroundings are predisposed to a

* Additional Professor, Department of ENT, PGI, Chandigarh.

variety of disorders which ranges from poor development of the child, skin problems, respiratory problem, gastrointestinal disorders and even the discharging ears. Recurrent upper respiratory tract infections in children predisposes them to ear infections in form of acute or chronic suppurative otitis media. This ear condition leads to hearing loss in the child which can be either conductive hearing loss that is usually reversible with treatment or sensorineural type of hearing loss which is a irreversible type of hearing loss. Hearing loss in childhood can also be either congenital or because of medications. Hearing loss in a child can directly affect his cognitive and speech development. Therefore, screening of all children for hearing is now recommended during infancy and early childhood so that they should have a normal speech and cognitive development. In adults besides chronic ear disorders various other significant factors related to one's lifestyle that causes hearing loss includes diseases like hypertension, diabetes mellitus, certain conditions like smoking, alcohol intake that leads to either direct affect on inner ear or affect the vestibulocochlear nerve or blood supply to the ear that in turn affects hearing. Noise trauma, i.e. exposure of ears to loud noises either single exposure to loud noise or repeated exposure to loud noises or continuous exposure to sound at workplaces can also leads to sensorineural type of hearing loss in certain group of people. Avoidance of working at high risk places or use of ear protection is advised to such people along with regular hearing assessments so as to predict damage to ears at an early stage and to prevent ears from further damage.

Repeated cleaning of ones ears with sticks/buds or unsterile objects by certain people causes trauma to the external ear canal which later on gets secondary infection and causes condition known as Otitis externa, which presents with pain, boil, discharge from ear and hearing loss. In these conditions simply avoiding such ear trauma and use of proper technique of ear cleaning can prevent these disorders.

People exposed to infected water especially during swimming leads to a condition called Swimmer's ears, that leads to infection of the external ear canal which manifests as ear blockade, pain, hearing loss and even ear discharge.

Avoidance of such pollutants and the use of ear protection during swimming is the best way to get rid of such painful conditions.

A condition in children known as strep throat also known as sorethroat or scratch throat is a bacterial infection in which child presents with fever, swollen lymph glands, abdominal pain for which the child requires repeated courses of medications. This condition is linked to poor hygiene and poor living conditions. There is increased incidence of tuberculosis in people living in unhealthy conditions. This condition, i.e. tuberculosis may present with simple neck swellings, i.e. cervical lymphadenopathy or voice disorders, i.e. tubercular laryngitis or hearing loss with ear discharge, i.e. tuberculous otitis media. Timely diagnosis and proper medication can prevent all the complications of this disorders that can at times be very troublesome.

Timely diagnosis, improving personal hygiene and proper treatment alongwith improvement in dietary intake, i.e. proper nutrition is the key to avoiding some of the serious complications which these diseases could lead to in all age groups.

Exposure of individuals to certains allergens like pollens, molds, animal danders, dust, certain food products can lead to a variety of allergic manifestations which affects most of systems in our body. Presentation of these allergies can be in form of simple itching in nose, eyes, ears, throat, sneezing, rhinorrhea (watering from nose), watering from eyes, irritating cough, to diseases like bronchial asthma and atopic dermatitis. In nose repeated exposures to allergens can lead to diseases like chronic sinusitis and nasal polyposis that might present as chronic nasal discharge and nasal obstruction. This nasal discharge can be source of constant discomfort to the person as repeated cleaning of one's throat is required. Nasal obstruction which is usually bilateral can cause a lot of discomfort to the person in form of compulsary oral or mouth breathing and sleep disturbances. Allergies can also affect the vocal cords and larynx of a person and can lead to voice change and also predisposes a person to recurrent laryngeal infections.

Avoidance of allergen exposure is always indicated

although it may be difficult to achieve. Measures that help control indoor allergen exposure include placement of dust proof covers over pillowes and mattresses, frequent dusting of surfaces and floors with a damp mop, maintenance of an indoor humidity below 50% and avoidance or frequent bathing of indoor pets if the patient is sensitive to animals. Measures that help control outdoor allergens include closing of windows, running of air conditioners and avoidance of lawn mowing and leaf raking. All this can make one's life free of such irritating manifestations that affect day-to-day activities and performance of an individual.

Poor oral hygiene and bad eating habits lead to an array of oral cavity disorders that affect the food intake of an individual and interferes with normal living. Lack of regular brushing of teeth, improper rinsing of mouth after food intake, excessive intake of sweets like chocolates especially during bedtime, chewing of tobacco and smoking can lead to reduction of normal microflora, leading to increase in the counts of harmful mico-organisms in mouth, that further leads to increase in anaerobic organism and more decaying material in oral cavity. This can present as foul smell from oral cavity and can also lead to decaying of teeth, i.e. dental caries. Smoking can stain the teeth, chewing of beetel nut and pan can lead to development of pre-cancerous condition like sub-mucous fibrosis in oral cavity can even or lead to oral cancer formation. Various dietary deficiencies like vitamin and mineral deficiencies or some systemic disorders especially gastrointestinal diseases can also lead to presentation like aphthous ulcers in oral cavity, stomatitis, cheilitis that causes pain while taking ones food and decreases food intake and can even interferes with perception of taste.

Avoidance of bad foods, e.g. sweets, alcohol, tobacco, beetel nuts along with intake of balanced food that included all vitamins—mineral with timely care of systemic disorders and proper oral cavity cleaning with regular oral cavity check-ups can make ones life relatively free of these disturbing conditions.

It is thought that increased exposure of an individual to cigarette smoke and alcohol intake predisposes that person to development of malignancies presenting in oral cavity and throat especially laryngeal cancers. Though research is still going on to find out various other aetiological factors for development of laryngeal malignancies, including genetic predisposition of an individual to oral and laryngeal cancers but alcohol and smoking is still thought to be the commonest cause. Although with advances in the management of these cancers over a period of time and with better rehabilitative procedures after surgery or radiotherapy, there is still a lot of psychological and financial burden on the individual after treatment. Thus, it is always better that if we could reduce the prevalence of the disease by avoiding the predisposing factors, i.e. avoidence of smooking and alcohol intake.

Improper use of our voice and excessive use of voice like in professional singers, teachers or people in marketing profession who have to phonate more as compared to other people are at increased risk of having vocal cord disorders like vocal cord nodule formation. This develops due to excessive and inappropriate use of ones voice. Vocal hygiene, i.e. use of speech in a proper way is important in our day-to-day life, so that we have a good voice for rest of our life.

Last but not the least obesity which is a gift of modern lifestyle to us affects the nasal passage and oral cavity of people, along with predisposing one to problems like hypertension, diabetes, coronary artery diseases, etc. These people presents with complaints like snoring, nasal obstruction, inability to sleep during night, day-time sleepiness, decreased in concentration and work performance. This can manifest in a bigger way like sleep apnea syndrome, pulmonary hypertension and right heart failure. All this can be avoided by simply reducing the weight of a person and changing ones lifestyle which includes dietary changes and increased physical activity.

Thus, it is important for us to understand that our surroundings and our lifestyle has tremendous effect on our body and our health. That is why it becomes all the more important for us to known that we should modify our lifestyle accordingly so as to have a healthy and cheerful life.

11

HOLISTIC HEALING

RANJIV MITTAL*

The relationship between thinking and health/disease has been the subject for speculation since the birth of modern medicine. Initially body and mind were considered separate entities with rigid compartmentalization of diseases. Over a period of time the influence of one over the other was recognized both in health and causation of disease and the concept of psychosomatic diseases was born. In the beginning psychic influence over soma and *vice versa* was limited to small area. Gradually the influence of emotions became noticeable in other areas as well. The evidence is becoming so compelling that now body and mind is considered a single entity, the mind being the invisible part of body and body the visible part of mind. Some of the studies mentioned below highlighted some of the psychosocial factors in the causation of disease process.

* Private Consultant, Holistic Healing, Sector 35, Chandigarh.

THE HARVARD MASTERY STRESS STUDY

Students were asked to describe their relationship to mother and father as:

1. Very close,
2. Warm and friendly,
3. Tolerant, and
4. Strained and cold

Thirty-five years later medical records revealed amazing results. 91% of participants who did not perceive themselves to have had a warm relationship with their mother had serious diagnosed diseases in mid-life (including coronary artery disease, high blood pressure, duodenal ulcer and alcoholism) as compared to only 45% of those who perceived themselves to have had warm relationship with their mothers. Similarly, 82% of participants who had low warmth and closeness scores with their fathers had diagnosed diseases in mid-life compared to only 50% of those who had high warmth and closeness scores with their fathers.

All 100% of participants who rated both their mothers and fathers low in warmth and closeness thirty-five years earlier had diseases diagnosed mid-life. Only 47% of those who rated both their fathers and mothers high in warmth and closeness had diagnosed diseases in mid-life.

JOHNS HOPKINS STUDY

1100 male medical students in 1940's assessed the quality of their relationship with their parents. It was found that doctors who subsequently developed cancers, committed suicide, had to be hospitalized for mental illness had suffered more from loneliness and interpersonal difficulties one to fifty years earlier.

The Scotland Study, the Durkheim Study and other studies have reached the same conclusion. Between 1979 and 1994 eight large-scale community-based studies were conducted. Although there was a lot of variation in these communities—from California to Eastern Finland, from

Georgia to Sweden—as well as differences in how social support and social isolation were measured, these studies showed remarkably consistent results.

Those who were socially isolated had at least two to five times the risk of premature death from all causes when compared to those who had a strong sense of connection and community.

THE ALAMEDA COUNTY STUDY

It was found that those who lacked social and community ties were more likely (1.9 to 3.1 times) to die during the nine-year follow-up. Almost seven thousand men and women participated in this study. The relationship between social ties, stage of disease, and survival was analyzed in a subset of 525 black and 486 white women in Alameda city with newly diagnosed breast cancer. Both black and white women reporting few sources of emotional support had almost twice the death rate from breast cancer during the five-year period of follow-up.

The Tecumseh study, The Swedish studies, The Finland study, The Evans county study, The three communities study, all reach the same conclusions.

THE BETA-BLOCKER HEART ATTACK TRIAL

In this study 2300 men who had survived a heart attack were interviewed. Those who were classified as being socially isolated and having a high degree of life stress had four times the risk of death as compared to men who had low levels of both stress and isolation even when controlling for other prognostic factors such as genetics, smoking, diet, alcohol, exercise, weight, and so on. This risk of death applied both to total deaths and sudden cardiac deaths. These psychological factors had a much more powerful effect on premature deaths than did the beta-blocker drug being tested. Ironically beta-blockers are being widely prescribed by cardiologists while psychosocial factors are often ignored.

The interesting part is that these factors are more important than those already being highlighted by modern medicine like smoking, alcohol, diet, exercise and medicines/ drugs. The reversal of this so-called lifestyle and thinking is capable of not only halting the disease process at any stage but reverse it in many instances both at individual level and in population studies. The under mentioned studies are providing indisputable evidence.

BELIEFS: PATHWAYS TO HEALTH AND WELL-BEING

My mother had a reoccurrence of cancer breast that had metastasized to her skull, spine, ribs and pelvis. The doctors gave her a poor prognosis and basically said they would do what they could to make her comfortable.

My mother and I spent four long days working with her beliefs about herself and her illness. As a result of the work we did with her beliefs, she was able to make dramatic improvements in her health elected not to have chemotherapy, radiation treatment, or any other traditional therapy. Seven years later, she is in excellent health and there have been no further cancer symptoms She swims one half-mile several times per week and is living a happy full life that includes trips to Europe and roles in TV commercials. She is an inspiration for all of us about what is possible for people with life-threatening illnesses.—*Robert Dilts*

ASTHMA FREE IN 21 DAYS—BY KATHRYN SHAFER

November 6, 1996. It is the morning of the New York City Marathon. I dress in running gear. At 10:45 A.M. twenty-nine thousand runners begin 2 miles marathon race. I am runner 26948, woman 6806—me an asthmatic since the age of fifteen months. Suddenly moments from my past come flooding back. My life spent in hospital rooms, under oxygen tents, taking frequent doses of inhalers and tablets shots flashed before me. Till the age of twenty-five I was on anti-asthmatic medicine. Then I started Healing Visualisations with Dr. Epstein. In next 21 days I felt the difference. Now I have completed one of world's most famous marathon without any anti-asthmatic medicines.

LEAN ON ME INTERVENTION STUDIES

In 1989 David Spiegel and colleagues at Stanford Medical School published a landmark article in *The Lancet* in which they studied women with metastatic breast cancer. His intention was to disprove the idea that psychosocial interventions could prolong the life of women with breast cancer. Dr. Spiegel wrote: "Our follow-up study was to investigate whether psychosocial intervention, which significantly reduced anxiety, depression, and pain, would do so without having any effect on the course of the disease."

In this study women with metastatic breast cancer were randomly assigned to two groups. Both groups received conventional medical care such as chemotherapy, surgery, and radiation. In addition, one group of women met together for ninety minutes once a week for a year. Patients were encouraged to come regularly and to express their feelings about the illness and its effect on their lives in a supportive environment that felt safe enough for them to express what they were really feeling—including their fears of disfigurement, of dying, of being abandoned by their friends and spouse, and so on. The group was led by a psychiatrist or a social worker plus a therapist who had breast cancer in remission. As a result, a strong sense of intimacy developed and these women began to love and care for each other. Five years later Dr. Spiegel studied the data. These women who had the social support group lived on an average twice as long as did the other group of women who did not have the support group.

In a related study, Dr. F.I. Fawzy and colleagues at the UCLA School of medicine published an article in 1993 evaluating reoccurrence and survival in patients with malignant melanoma who had participated in a six-week intervention five to six years earlier. Patients whose malignant melanoma was surgically removed were randomly assigned to support group or to a comparison group. None of the patients in either group received any kind of conventional treatment other than surgery. The results were similar to Dr. Spiegel study.

LOVE AND SURVIVAL—BY DEAN ORNISH

I am not aware of any other factor in medicine—not diet, not smoking, not exercise, not stress, not genetics, not drugs, not surgery—that has a greater impact on our quality of life, incidence of illness, and premature death from all causes. That power is that of Love and Intimacy.

Dr. Dean Ornish conducted a study, which he has published in a book entitled Reversal of the Heart Disease. Participants were asked to make changes in five areas of their lives. These areas are:

1. Diet,
2. Exercise,
3. Opening your heart to your own self,
4. Opening your heart to others, and
5. Opening your heart to a higher self.

Computerized angiographic studies done after one year of lifestyle changes were compared with those done in the beginning of study. The results were astounding. The coronary arteries had started opening up in 92% of the patients.

Love medicine and Miracles—By Bernie Siegal, Anatomy of an illness—By Norman Coussins are couple of other internationally reputed workers in this area whose work with self and others is a landmark in mind-body medicine.

Why then we the trained men of medicine the healers, are not able to take this hard core evidence into consideration and achieve more flexibility? We are ready to prescribe medicines at a much more flimsy evidence. Oral serratopeptidase! Has any body seen the study of effectiveness of this drug in human beings but this is selling like hot peanuts. The reasons to my mind are basically two—

1. The influence of drug companies which are directing most of research in medicine.
2. Our own perception that thinking is very difficult to change and no tools are available.

Most of the research conducted these days is funded by

drug companies and naturally these corporate giants are going to keep their own interests in mind. We are fed ready-made information about the effectivity of drugs without informing about alternate ways of healing which might be effective without the risk of side effects.

Lifestyle changes are easy to make. Tools are there with us since long, only requirement is to learn these methods with the same sincerity as we learn about drugs and apply them with full confidence on ourselves and others. Some of these tools are progressive muscular relaxation, creative visualization, directed visualization, neuro linguistic programming, hypnosis, time line therapy and so on.

12

CANCER NEWS AND TRENDS

1. Fiber Overload Won't Stop Recurring Colon Polyps (Health Scout News—05/11/2002)

Don't toss your All-Bran yet, but new research shows that fiber intake did not affect the recurrence rate of colon polyps. All the participants entering the trial were already consuming higher-than-average amounts of fiber, however, which may have skewed the results. "Because they were already consuming fiber, they may already have been protected," says Elizabeth Jacobs, lead author of the study appearing in the *Journal of the National Cancer Institute.*

Colon cancer, the second biggest cancer killer in the United States, starts with tiny polyps in the colon. Plenty of evidence suggests that the cancer is at least partially caused by environmental factors. And anecdotal evidence suggests that high-fiber diets may protect against the cancer. The ideal study, Jacobs adds, would look at what people eat through their entire lives, because it takes at least 10 to 20 years for colorectal cancer to develop. Such a study, however, is unlikely to occur. Another important area for research is to determine where intake is most important: for prevention or to slow down growth rates of the polyps. Still, Jacobs says, none of this means you should stop eating fiber, especially given that it seems to have beneficial effects on other aspects of health, such as heart disease and diabetes.

2. Unstable Chromosomes Could Kick Off Colon Cancer (Reuters Health—18/11/2002)

A mutation in a gene called APC is believed to be present in most cases of colorectal cancer, but new research raises the possibility that a defective APC gene may not be the first step on the road to cancer. Unlike that age-old question, though, determining whether changes in APC or unstable chromosomes come first could have important implications for cancer therapy, according to Lengauer. Documenting the first step in colorectal cancer, he said, will give scientists a target for developing new treatments to destroy cancer in its earliest stages, before it has a chance to spread. In about 85% of the cases, the APC gene is defective in colorectal cancer. This gene helps regulate the growth of cells, so if it is not working properly, cancer cells can grow unchecked. To develop new therapies for colorectal cancer, it is important to know what the earliest steps in the cancer process are, Lengauer said. If changes in APC come first, then it might be possible to develop a drug to prevent those changes, he said. Alternately, a drug that keeps chromosomes stable might stave-off cancer if chromosomal instability is the initial step in colorectal cancer, according to Lengauer. The model does not prove that chromosomal instability is the first step, but it does give researchers a starting point, he said.

3. Common Virus May be Linked to Colorectal Cancer (Health Scout News—15/11/2002)

A virus that lurks harmlessly in the bodies of tens of millions of Americans may play a role in the development of colorectal cancer, new research suggests. The findings are preliminary, and the germ—known as human cytomegalovirus (CMV)—might not actually contribute to the development of the second deadliest type of cancer, says study co-author Dr. Charles S. Cobbs. Colorectal cancer is "notoriously difficult to treat," Cobbs says, especially if it spreads to other organs such as the liver. Colorectal cancer typically strikes people over the age of 50. Screening tests are available, and experts estimate that they could detect and prevent 90 percent of the cases.

Cobbs says his investigation into colorectal cancer was inspired by his previous research into the possible role that human cytomegalovirus (CMV) could play in brain tumors.

CMV is a type of herpes virus, a member of the same family of germs that cause cold sores, genital herpes, chicken pox, some kinds of mononucleosis and Epstein-Barr virus. Except for infants, who can be especially vulnerable, the virus almost never causes symptoms. "It's thought to lie around latent in the body and not do anything," Cobbs says. The exceptions are people with weak immune systems, such as AIDS patients, and those who are on special drugs because of organ transplants. CMV is extremely common in Third World countries, where close to 100 percent of the population may be infected. The virus is transmitted through saliva and urine, Myers says. Breastfeeding can transmit the disease, says Cobbs, and so can sex. Gay men are especially at high risk. However, previous research suggests CMV could pave the way for the development of cancer in the body, he adds. Researchers are working on vaccines, though, and some drugs do treat the infection.

4. New Link to Colon Cancer Found (Health Scout News—02/12/2002)

A common human virus may be associated with colon cancer. So says a study in the *Journal Cancer Research*. Temple University researchers say they found evidence that the JC virus (JCV) may play a role in development of intestinal tract tumors. JCV infects more than 90 percent of humans, usually during early childhood. It most likely infects people through the upper respiratory tract and remains latent in most people throughout their lives. However, in some people with weakened immune systems, JCV can become active and may cause brain cancer. Along with infecting people through the upper respiratory tract, JCV may get into people through contaminated food and water. That takes the virus into different areas of the body, including the intestinal tract. The researchers found genetic evidence of JCV in samples of large intestine tumors. However, more research is needed to determine if JCV actually causes those tumors or plays a different role.

5. New Tests May Detect Early Signs of Cancers (Reuters—29/10/2002)

A new test that detects a group of molecules in cancerous cells could revolutionize cancer screening by picking up early signs of bowel, cervical and other common forms of the disease. Professor Ron Laskey of the University of Cambridge and his colleagues have developed a simple, non-invasive test that pinpoints a group of molecules called MCMs which are found in rapidly dividing cancerous cells but not in healthy cells. If further studies confirm the results of early trials, he believes the molecular markers could form the basis for screening tests for bowel and other types of cancer such as cervical, bladder, oral, lung and breast. "It is affordable, non-invasive and it has the potential to revolutionize cancer screening," Nobel Prize winner Sir Paul Nurse told a science conference. Nurse, the chief executive of the Medical Charity Cancer Research, UK, added that Laskey's work is an example of how understanding the basic biology of cell division can produce a test to detect cancer.

Bowel cancer is one of the most common cancers but if it is detected and treated early, the survival rates are high. Laskey believes the test could form the basis for a screening program for the disease, along with a bowel examination, by detecting the molecules in samples of feces. "We're really excited by our results so far, which suggests that our test is not only sensitive but also specific, in that it does not accidentally pick out healthy people as having bowel cancer," he added.

6. Women Should Start Colon Cancer Screening at 50 (Reuters Health—21/10/2002)

Even though research has suggested that women may develop colorectal cancer at an older age than men, findings presented at the American College of Gastroenterology's annual meeting do not support beginning screening later in life in women. "The current guidelines recommend screening to begin at age 50 in an average-risk person," lead author Dr. Brooks D. Cash of the Uniformed Services University of the Health Sciences in Bethesda, Maryland, told Reuters Health. Cash and colleagues sought to discover if this screening recommendation is appropriate for both men and women.

"This analysis essentially breaks down prevalence according to age, in an effort to determine if the appropriate screening age for colon cancer in women is later or the same (as) in men," he said.

7. One Bad Copy of Gene Boosts Colon Cancer Risk (Reuters Health—20/09/2002)

A gene mutation found in people of Ashkenazi Jewish descent appears to boost colorectal cancer risk, according to a report. Scientists already knew the gene defect causes Bloom syndrome, a rare cancer-susceptibility condition that occurs when both copies of the gene—one inherited from each parent—are defective. The new study suggests that people who inherit one healthy copy and one mutated copy of the gene have two to three times the risk of developing colorectal cancer as people without the gene mutation. "The main finding of our study is that a genetic mutation found in about 1 in 120 people of Ashkenazi Jewish descent causes colorectal cancer," said the study's lead author Dr. Stephen B. Gruber, during an interview with Reuters Health. "We estimate that this one genetic alteration accounts for somewhere between 1% to 2% of all colorectal cancer among Ashkenazi Jews," said Gruber, of the University of Michigan Medical School in Ann Arbor. The gene is called BLM and two studies of the gene—one in mice and one in humans—are published in the *Journal Science.*

8. Radiation Alone Can Treat Rectal Cancer (Health Scout News—06/09/2002)

Radiation therapy alone is adequate treatment for people with rectal cancer who don't want surgery or can't have it because they're in poor physical shape. So says a new study that appears in the *International Journal of Radiation Oncology, Biology and Physics.*

Surgery is the most common treatment for rectal cancer. It's sometimes combined with radiation therapy to improve the outcome. However, some people can't have surgery because they're in poor physical condition. Others won't consent to surgery and its possible side effects. "Surgery remains, without a doubt, the main treatment of rectal adenocarcinoma. Nevertheless, in inoperable patients, combined radiation therapy should be considered," says study author Dr. Jean-Pierre Gerard of the Centre Antoine-Lacassagne in France. "Research aimed at improving the quality of life of patients with rectal cancer is ongoing, and this study contributes to that body of knowledge," he says.

9. Scientists Find Clue to Bowel Cancer Survival (Reuters Health—03/09/2002)

Scientists said they had found a gene that appears to play a key role in determining patients' chances of surviving bowel cancer. The team, at the University Hospital of Basel in Switzerland, said that patients were three times more likely to benefit from chemotherapy if their tumors tested positive for the gene. Detecting the gene—called SMAD4—could help doctors to predict whether chemotherapy will work, allowing them to tailor treatments to individual patients needs. The scientists were interested to see whether it could also affect the success of chemotherapy. They analyzed tumor samples from 202 patients with bowel cancer who had been treated with standard chemotherapy, including the drug 5-fluorouracil. In healthy bowel tissue, each cell usually has two copies of the SMAD4 gene. The researchers found that patients whose cancer cells had both copies of the gene were three times more likely to remain free of the disease following chemotherapy than those whose tumors had lost at least one of their copies. In two-thirds of patients, at least one copy of the gene was missing from their tumors.

10. New Pain Meds Treat Spread of Colon Cancer in Mice (Reuters Health—15/08/2002)

COX-2 inhibitors, a newer class of painkillers designed to circumvent side effects associated with older drugs, may also treat colon cancer that has spread to the liver, according to new study findings. Nobuya Yamada of the Osaka City University Graduate School of Medicine in Japan and colleagues found that giving COX-2 to mice with colon cancer that had spread to their livers shrank the animals' liver tumors. In addition, when they added the COX-2 inhibitor to a Petri dish containing a strain of colon cancer cells, the researchers found that the treatment prevented the multiplication and spread of the malignant cells. Based on these results, Yamada told Reuters Health that he and his colleagues suspect that COX-2 inhibitors may help prevent the recurrence of cancer that has spread to the liver. "We recommend patients with colon cancer to take COX-2 inhibitors after surgical (removal of part of the) colon," Yamada said.

11. Eloxatin to Treat Colon Cancer (Health Scout News—13/08/2002)

In the fastest review ever, the U.S. Food and Drug Administration has approved the use of a drug to fight colon cancer, the nation's second-leading cause of cancer death. Eloxatin is a last-ditch treatment, to be used when all other treatment options have failed. And its success rate hasn't been stellar. Only 9 percent of patients who received the drug had their tumors shrink measurably. Even then, the treatment was good only for about two months, when the tumors resumed their growth. That's the not-so-good news. The hopeful news is that the clinical trials were performed on patients who were hard-to-treat and had exhausted other chemotherapy.

The FDA anticipates that results from ongoing trials may show that Eloxatin will work better when administered when colon cancer is at an earlier stage. Dr. Richard Pazdur, who heads up the FDA's cancer research, stressed that the agency is willing to work around the clock to find whether a drug is suitable when lives are at stake. "We want to send a message," Pazdur told the Associated Press, emphasizing that FDA employees worked overtime and cancelled vacations to speedily review Eloxatin because the science behind the drug was so strong. "We're willing to do that if we think the drug is worth that."

12. Super Side Effects (Daily News—04/08/2002)

In his lab at Weill Cornell Medical College, Dr. Andrew Dannenberg studies Celebrex, one of two hugely popular arthritis pain drugs. But his interest is different: Can its main ingredient, COX-2, fight cancer? The answer is yes. Studies show that the COX-2 inhibitor in Celebrex reduces growth of pre-cancerous polyps in a rare form of colon cancer so well that the pills are now approved by the Food and Drug Administration for that purpose. "That medications may have secondary benefits is underappreciated by many health-care providers as well as patients," said Dannenberg, who heads cancer prevention at Weill Cornell Medical Center.

Statins, the powerful cholesterol-lowering drugs that are revolutionizing cardiac care, are being studied as potential treatments for osteoporosis, bone loss, Alzheimer's disease and cancer.

A cancer drug, methotrexate, has become, in small doses, "the gold standard" for treating wickedly painful rheumatoid arthritis, Cronstein said.

13. Scientists Find New Clues About How Cancer Spreads (Reuters—05/08/2002)

Scientists have discovered how a key protein helps cancerous cells spread through the body in a finding that could pave the way for new drugs to slow the progression of the disease. The molecule, called Src, loosens the tissue around a tumor and allows cancerous cells to metastasize, or grow in other organs. Scientists at Glasgow's Beatson Institute, who figured out how it works, believe drugs designed to block the action of the molecule could prevent cancer from spreading. "We discovered what it is actually doing in human cancer cells. It is important in the molecular understanding of how cancer cells spread," Professor Margaret Frame, who headed the research team, said.

"Hopefully we can slow down the disease in patients," Frame added. She is confident that drugs that either prevent the cancer from spreading from the original tumor or slow down its progression if it has already started could be developed in the next few years. "Improving our understanding of how cancer spreads should help in the development of drugs to block the process," she said. "If we could confine cancer cells to the original tumor it would give surgery a much greater chance of success and reduce the risk of the disease reappearing in other parts of the body."

14. Growth Hormone Tied to Colon Cancer (Health Scout News—25/07/2002)

Human growth hormone, which is given to children and adults to make up for deficits in natural levels of the substance, just might increase the risk of colon cancer decades later. A new British study, appearing in The Lancet, showed a statistically significant increase in colorectal cancer among people who took non-synthetic pituitary growth hormone between 1959 and 1985. However, the absolute number of cancer cases was small, and researchers say there's no proven biological reason for such a link, if it's indeed real. They also note that, since the mid-1980s, doctors have been prescribing a synthetic form of growth hormone that may have different effects on the body. What's more, doctors now administer the drug at doses designed not to exceed age-appropriate thresholds, and patients are carefully monitored to make sure their blood levels of the substance stay in this range.

Before 1985, the substance was pulled from the pituitary glands of cadavers and was prone to contamination, Melmed explains. "We just don't know what those impurities were" or what, if any, harm they might have caused, he says. Today's synthetic growth hormone is not only pristine, but it's administered in strictly controlled doses that stay within the normal range, he adds. Moreover, although growth hormone can cause tumors to grow faster, there's no evidence that it causes them to appear. A large study of people with acromegaly, whose excessive growth hormone production causes them to become giants, found no increase in the risk of cancer, Melmed says.

15. Folate Supplement May Reduce Colon Cancer Risk (Reuters Health—18/07/2002)

Findings from a small UK study suggest that taking a folate supplement daily could help ward-off colon cancer in people at risk of the disease. Previous research has suggested that taking folate supplements, or eating a folate-rich diet, could help reduce the risk of this type of cancer. While folate, a B vitamin also known as folic acid, is found in fruit and green, leafy vegetables and frequently added to grains including bread and cereal, it can also be taken in supplement form. Colon cancer is one of the most common cancers and often develops over several years from small growths called polyps. In the current investigation, lead author K. Khosraviani of Royal Victoria Hospital in Belfast, Northern Ireland, and colleagues evaluated the effects of a 2-milligram supplement of folate, taken each day for 3 months, in six people with recurrent colon polyps. They were compared with five people who also had recurrent polyps but took an inactive placebo instead. All of the men and women in the study had tissue samples from their rectums analyzed before, during and after the study period.

16. More Aggressive Colon Cancer Screening Urged (Health Scout News—15/07/2002)

More evidence that early screening reduces death from colon cancer has prompted a government group to boost its recommendation that everyone over 50 be screened for the disease. The U.S. Preventive Services Task Force (USPSTF) has given its highest level, "A," recommendation to health-care professionals to test people over 50 for colon cancer, up from a "B" recommendation in 1996, says Dr. Paul S. Frame, a member of the task force. "The level of evidence has increased since 1996, from one to four randomized studies showing that a fecal occult blood test is effective is reducing mortality from colon cancer, and the data is pretty much the same for sigmoidoscopies," he says.

Data showing that colonoscopies are also an effective test was convincing as well, he adds. People at a higher risk for the disease, like those with a family history, should be tested at younger ages, Frame says. But because 90 percent of colon cancers appear in people over age 50, that's a good age to start undergoing screenings, he says. The recommendations appear in the Annals of Internal Medicine.

The fecal occult test, for instance, is simple, can be done at home and has the most evidence that it reduces mortality, Frame says, but since what you are testing for is blood in the stool rather than cancer, there are a lot of false positives because there are other reasons you can have blood in your stool. A sigmoidoscopy is effective because it presents a visual picture of the colon so a doctor can clearly see the polyps that might be cancerous, but the procedure only looks at the lower part of the colon, and there is some discomfort with the procedure.

17. New Stool-Based Colorectal Cancer Screen Promising (Reuters Health—31/05/2002)

A new stool-based screening test to detect colorectal cancer has shown encouraging results, according to preliminary study findings. In a small group of patients, the test detected 37 out of 40 people with cancer—including 9 cases of early, highly curable disease—and designated all 25 healthy people as cancer-free. The new test "does appear to be highly discriminating between normal patients and patients with cancer," lead author Dr. Nicholas Coleman of the Hutchison/MRC Research Centre in Cambridge, UK, told Reuters Health.

18. Keyhole Surgery Better for Colon Cancer-Study (Reuters Health—28/06/2002)

Spanish surgeons recommended keyhole surgery for colon cancer patients, saying it can reduce complications and prolong cancer-free survival. Keyhole surgery, or laparoscopy-assisted colectomy (LAC), is less invasive than normal surgery and also shortens hospital stays and lessens the chances of a recurrence of the cancer. Instead of normal surgery, LAC involves tiny incisions and the insertion of a small camera to enable surgeons to see and remove the tumour. "Our results show that LAC should be preferred to open colectomy in patients with colon cancer," said Dr. Antonio Lacy of the Hospital Clinic in Barcelona.

19. Veggies Slow Spread—Not Start—Of Colon Cancer (Reuters Health—21/06/2002)

Eating relatively high levels of fruits and vegetables appears unlikely to prevent development of polyps, the initially harmless abnormalities in the intestine that can eventually develop into colon cancer, according to new research. Previous studies of vegetable intake and colon cancer have found that eating fruits and vegetables can reduce the risk of the disease. But while eating well may not reduce the risk of developing polyps, it may stop potentially dangerous polyps from becoming cancer, according to study lead author Dr. John D. Potter of the Fred Hutchinson Cancer Research Center in Seattle, Washington.

20. Vitamin D's Cancer Protection Explained (Reuters Health—16/05/2002)

New research suggests that Vitamin D may protect against colon cancer by helping to get rid of a toxic acid that promotes the disease. The discovery could point the way to the development of therapies that provide the cancer protection of Vitamin D without the side effects caused by consuming too much of the vitamin, the study's lead author told Reuters Health in an interview. "Now we believe that we have discovered the potential mechanism of how Vitamin D can be protective of colon cancer," said Dr. David J. Mangelsdorf of the Howard Hughes Medical Institute at the University of Texas Southwestern Medical Center in Dallas. If it is not the only mechanism, it is "at least one of them," he said. Mangelsdorf explained that Vitamin D is known to protect against colon cancer, but exactly how has been uncertain.

The research also provides a possible explanation of how high-fat diets may increase the risk of colon cancer. Since LCA is released from the liver when a person eats fatty food, a high-fat diet that keeps LCA levels high may "overwhelm the system," Mangelsdorf said. He speculated that the body may stop producing enough CYP3A to keep LCA under control. He added that a high-fat diet is "something our bodies were never, never meant to have to deal with." The study does not prove that a high-fat diet increases the risk of colon cancer, according to Mangelsdorf, but "it gives us a testable hypothesis for testing the effects of a high-fat diet." The discovery may also help researchers develop drugs to prevent colon cancer. Too much Vitamin D can have harmful effects, but it may be possible to develop a drug that would provide the vitamin's cancer-protective effects without its harmful side effects.

21. Pope Helps Launch Global Anti-Cancer Effort (Reuters Health—25/03/2002)

Pope John Paul helped launch a campaign aiming to prevent millions of people from dying of cancers of the stomach and gut. Speaking to the organisers of the first global campaign against digestive cancers during an audience at the Vatican, the Pope gave his blessing to their endeavour. "His Holy Father underlined the importance not only of prevention, but also the need to train doctors to defeat one of the most serious illnesses to afflict mankind," Alberto Montori, professor of surgery at Rome University, said. "Screening for colorectal cancer and polyps should be offered to all men and women starting at age 50," Winawer said, adding that trials show screening significantly reduces mortality. The cost in terms of life-years saved, he said, is similar to mammography.

22. Calcium May Cut Risk of Colon Cancer (Health Scout News—10/03/2002)

Increasing your calcium intake may reduce the risk of cancer in the distal—or left side—of the colon. "We found that a moderate intake of 700 milligrams to 800 milligrams of calcium per day may decrease the risk of left-sided colon cancer in both men and women," says Dr. Kana Wu, lead author of what she calls a preliminary study, and a research fellow at Harvard University's School of Public Health. Individuals, who had the increased calcium in their diets showed a 40 percent to 50 percent lower risk of developing this type of colon cancer, compared with those who were taking less than 500 milligrams of calcium daily. Intakes higher than 700 or 800 milligrams, however, didn't show the same protective effect. In other words, there appeared to be a threshold or upper limit to the benefits. (Federal health officials recommend between 800 milligrams and 1,300 milligrams a day for adults, depending on your age and sex.) The researchers also found that the benefit from calcium could be enhanced by taking Vitamin D. "Vitamin D is important for absorption of calcium and these two nutrients are closely linked," Wu says. "If there is not enough Vitamin D, the calcium cannot be absorbed properly."

23. Value of UK Cancer Evaluation Rule Questioned (Reuters Health—19/03/2002)

Two years ago, the UK government issued an edict that patients with symptoms suggestive of certain types of upper gastrointestinal tract cancers be evaluated within 2 weeks. This so-called "2-week rule" is a hot topic at the Annual Scientific Meeting of the British Society of Gastroenterology under way in Birmingham, where the consensus seems to be that it is not effective and may even be counter-productive. According to one expert, the rule has actually wound up delaying treatment for patients whose cancer symptoms do not meet the "2-week rule" criteria. "It's an idea that's not really based on good scientific evidence that has really been pushed through more for political reasons."

24. New Test to Detect Colorectal Cancer Early (Times of India Online—27/01/2002)

Tracking and isolating a colon cancer-causing gene could be used to test patients for early signs of the disease, greatly improving their chances of a cure, according to a study published in the *New England Journal of Medicine.* In a oncological collaboration led by Bert Vogelstein of the Howard Hughes Medical Institute, researchers were able to successfully detect mutations in the cancer-causing APC gene in about 60 percent of early-stage colorectal cancer patients.

Eventually, the APC screen could be combined with another test that detects mutations in another gene known as BAT26, also isolated by Vogelstein's team, to together detect "over 80 per cent of (cancerous) lesions."

25. Researchers Caution on Colon Surgery (Times of India Online—16/01/2002)

A type of colon cancer surgery involving an extremely small incision does not necessarily mean a quicker, less painful recovery, and should be avoided until more is known about whether it helps people live longer, disease-free lives, researchers say. Laparoscopy, as this keyhole approach is called, is an increasingly common technique in many types of surgery. Laparoscopies require much smaller surgical openings, often resulting in speedier recoveries. Researchers led by Drs Jane Weeks of the Dana-Farber Cancer Institute and Heidi Nelson of the Mayo Clinic looked at 428 patients randomly selected to have colon cancer laparoscopies or traditional "open" surgery. Laparoscopy patients required only slightly less pain medication while hospitalized and were sent home, on average, just under a day earlier.

Both techniques require removing the tumor with a portion of the colon and sewing the rest back together, which may explain why there was little difference in quality-of-life measures, said Dr Ted Trimble of the National Cancer Institute, which helped fund the study. Nelson said the continuing study will examine the long-term effects of the procedure, and results may be seen in two to three years.

26. Study Okays Chemo for Elderly (Times of India Online—12/10/2001)

Elderly people with colon cancer can benefit from chemotherapy after surgery as much as younger patients can, and the side effects are no worse, a study found. The older you get, the greater the chance of colon cancer. But some doctors are reluctant to prescribe chemotherapy for patients over 65. For that matter, older patients may not want to take on six months of possible nausea, diarrhea and other side effects. "Older people will sometimes say, 'I'm not sure I'll save enough years of life to make that worth it to me,'" said Dr. Richard Goldberg, a cancer specialist at the Mayo Clinic in Rochester, Minn., and one of the authors. "What this study says is, 'If you're among the more robust sexagenarians or octogenarians, we can give you data to say that it will.'" Older patients generally tolerated chemotherapy as well as younger ones. Overall, chemotherapy increased the five-year survival rate from 64 percent to 71 percent, with no significant difference from age group to age group.

27. Popular Test Misses 76% of Colon Tumors: Study (Times of India Online—23/08/2001)

A widely used screening test for colon cancer misses 76 percent of suspicious growths and when combined with another test fails to detect 24 percent of tumors, researchers reported in a new study of the deadly disease that is highly treatable if caught in time.

The simplest of the two tests, called a fecal occult-blood test, looks for traces of blood in the feces that has been shed by tumors or by polyps that may grow into cancerous tumors. In tests on 2,885 volunteers, a research team led by Dr. David Liberman of the Portland VA Medical Center in Oregon found the fecal occult-blood test missed 76 percent of suspicious growths. Alternatively, when doctors directly examined the colon with a hollow tube known as a sigmoidoscope, 30 percent of the tumors, or pre-cancerous polyps, were missed, in part because the tube can only view the lower half of the colon. When the tests were combined, 24 percent of the growths were missed. Based on the new findings, "it seems logical that we should advocate colonoscopy for the screening of people without symptoms," said Dr. Allan S. Detsky of the University of Toronto, in an editorial in the Journal. "When adequate resources are available, colonoscopy is a better one-time screening test," Detsky said.

28. FDA Approves Camera-in-a-Pill (Times of India Online—03/08/2001)

Medicine has caught up with Hollywood: The government approved a tiny camera-in-a-capsule that patients can swallow to give doctors a close-up view of their small intestine. The camera painlessly winds its way through the digestive tract, using wireless technology to beam back colour pictures of the gut. The video pill is made by Israel-based Given Imaging Ltd. and called the M2A Swallowable Imaging Capsule. It's reminiscent of that sci-fi classic *Fantastic Voyage,* where a microscopic medical submarine is injected into the body.

"It's very sci-fi, and initially when the people from Given approached me two years ago I didn't believe it" could work, said Dr. Blair Lewis of New York's Mount Sinai School of Medicine, who tested the video pill on 20 patients and determined it works. "I have been shown to be wrong, it is believable and shows tremendous promise," Lewis said, estimating that many of some 25,000 people with internal bleeding of undiagnosed causes might be candidates to try the video pill.

A study of 57 healthy people found the video pill can safely pass through the digestive tract. In a study of 20 patients, it was found 60 per cent effective in uncovering an intestinal abnormality compared with just 35 per cent of abnormalities diagnosed using a traditional endoscope. The FDA allowed such small studies of the video pill because it is similar to today's endoscopic cameras, just in pill form instead of mounted on a tube.

29. Medimmune Searching for a Winner (Cancer Info—17/07/2001)

Medimmune Inc. of Gaithersburg said that it has launched trials of an experimental drug called Vitaxin in cancer patients. The two-part trial will first study the treatment in 16 patients with advanced cancer of the colon to evaluate its safety and appropriate dosage. If successful, the company will then enroll 40 more cancer patients to test its ability to shrink tumors.

James F. Young, Medimmune's president of research and development, said in a statement that "colorectal cancer is an important therapeutic target for Vitaxin since there is still significant unmet medical need."

Vitaxin is one of five drugs Medimmune has in early human testing. Vitaxin is an antibody that has the potential to stop the growth of new blood vessels. The company believes it could be used to treat inflammatory diseases such as rheumatoid arthritis and restenosis as well as cancer. Last year, a more potent version of the original molecule was developed. In March, the company launched its first human tests, designed to evaluate its safety and dosage, in 24 patients with solid tumors resistant to other treatments.

30. Toxin that Slows Colon Cancer Growth (Times of India Online—09/07/2001)

A bacterial toxin better known for causing "Montezuma's revenge"—or traveller's diarrhoea—could be a potential treatment for colon cancer, researchers reported this week. The toxin fits a receptor on cancer cells like a lock fits a key, and apparently can slow the growth of the cancerous cells, although it does not kill them outright.

If the toxin, which is produced by E coli bacteria and mimics naturally-occurring molecules in the body, can do the same in human patients it might be a potential treatment for colorectal cancer, lead researcher Dr. Scott A. Waldman of Thomas Jefferson University in Philadelphia, Pennsylvania, explained in an interview. However, much more study is needed to determine if this is safe and effective in humans.

31. Study Links Processed Meat to Cancer (Times of India Online—24/06/2001)

Eating lots of preserved meats such as salami, bacon, cured ham and hot dogs could increase the risk of bowel cancer by 50 per cent, early results of a major new study have suggested. However, when it came to fresh red meat beef, lamb, pork and veal there seemed to be no link.

Previous studies have linked high meat intake to colorectal cancer, but almost all the studies grouped fresh and processed meats together. The latest findings come from an ongoing study experts say is the most reliable research into the influence of diet on cancer to date an investigation involving almost half a million people, from southern Greece to northern Norway.

However, that does not mean red meat has been cleared of suspicion, said Dr Arthur Schatzkin, chief of nutritional epidemiology at the US National Cancer Institute.

32. Tests on Cancer Drug Suspended (Times of Online—19/05/2001)

Two national studies of a widely used drug for colorectal cancer were suspended for new patients because the drug turned out to be more toxic than expected. Some doctors have viewed the five-year-old drug irinotecan, also known by the brand name Camptosar, as the most useful drug against advanced colorectal cancer in years. It is recommended as standard therapy in combination with other drugs. However, almost three times as many patients died taking the standard drug combination in the latest studies sponsored by the National Cancer Institute.

33. New Vaccine Promising in Fight against Colon Cancer (Times of India Online—16/05/2001)

A new vaccine to treat colorectal cancers using genetically-altered cells has shown promising results among patients in late stages of the disease. The vaccine, which helps boost the patient's immune system, was effective in helping produce dendritic cells—immune system indicator cells—which then targeted the cancerous cells. Cancerous cells have an over-abundance of a protein known as CEA that is diminished when "attacked" by the boosted dendritic cells. Among the 12 patients tested in the study, four displayed clinical improvement in their colorectal or lung cancer. In two patients, all tumors regressed, with one patient in remission for almost a year. None of the patients experienced side effects, a benefit that could be extended to patients suffering from lung and breast cancer. The study demonstrates that a protein expressed in common malignancies can be vaccinated against and may ultimately be applicable to many patients.

Colorectal cancer is second behind lung cancer in causing fatalities among US patients. Among annual cancer-related deaths, 10.2 per cent can be attributable to colorectal cancer.

34. Doctors Encouraged by Experimental Cancer Drug (Times of India Online—14/05/2001)

A precisely aimed new drug that blocks the tumor's ability to fuel its own growth is proving useful in terminally ill-patients, encouraging doctors that decades of research into cancer biology is finally paying-off. Doctors said they expect the medicine to become a standard treatment for colon cancer and probably other tumors as well.

The latest treatment, code-named IMC-C225, produced no cures, but it did shrink tumors by at least half in nearly one-quarter of patients with end-stage colon cancer. "In a population of patients where we would expect the response rate to be zero, this is incredibly exciting. It means a lot of new hope for people with this disease," said Dr. Leonard B. Saltz of Memorial Sloan-Kettering Cancer Center in New York City. Saltz presented the results of experimental use on 120 patients at a meeting in San Francisco of the American Society of

Clinical Oncology.

Some cancer cells produce large amounts of molecules called growth factors. These stick to the receptors, triggering the cells to divide. This way, the cancer stimulates itself to grow. But by covering up the receptor, the antibody breaks cancer's feedback loop. While this may not kill cancer by itself, doctors say it appears to make tumors more vulnerable to the effects of chemotherapy. The only common side effect of the treatment was an acne-like skin rash.

35. Age and Gender Influence Colon Cancer Risk (Times of India Online—15/04/2001)

Older individuals and men are more likely to develop polyps and tumors in the colon than are younger individuals and women. Though advancing age has long been associated with the development of colon and other cancers, little research has been done to explore the influence of gender on colon cancer risk. The investigators, therefore, used a national database of colonoscopy results to examine the possible link between age and gender and the risk of developing polyps or tumors in the colon and rectum.

36. Contraceptive Pill may be Answer for Bowel Cancer (Times of India—17/04/2001)

New research bolsters the theory that the female hormone estrogen might protect women from colorectal cancer. Italian scientists have found that women had about a 20 per cent lower chance of developing the disease if they used oral contraceptives. For a while now it has been suspected that estrogen in the pill could protect against bowel cancer and the latest research has gone some way to confirm this. The findings are similar to those of a recent study that suggested that hormone replacement therapy, or HRT, could protect women from colorectal cancer to the same degree. Over the last 20 years death rates from bowel cancer have dropped more in women than in men. Some scientists believe this could be partly due to estrogen found in oral contraceptives and hormone replacement therapy.

Regular screening after the age of 50, regular exercise and maintaining a healthy weight are considered the best ways to reduce the chances of developing colorectal cancer.

37. Bowel Cancer Risk 'may be inherited' (Cancer Info—04/04/2001)

Nearly a third of all bowel cancer cases could be inherited. Scientists said this could lead to a test to identify the people most at risk from the disease and improve their chances of early diagnosis and treatment. The Cancer Research Campaign (CRC) funded team found that 30% of people with bowel cancer appeared to have an inherited problem with repairing their genes—compared to just 9% of the general population. Cancer develops after cells suffer damage to their genes causing them to divide out of control and eventually form tumours. Scientists think that people with defects in their system could be more likely to develop bowel cancer.

38. Ursodiol may Lower Risk of Colon Cancer in Ulcerative Colitis Patients at High Risk (Cancer Info—17/01/2001)

Ursodiol, a medication that reduces colonic levels of deoxycholic acid, appears to lower the frequency of colonic dysplasia in patients with ulcerative colitis and primary sclerosing cholangitis.

The study assessed the impact of ursodiol use on the development of colonic dysplasia in 59 patients with ulcerative colitis and primary sclerosing cholangitis. All patients were enrolled in a colonoscopic surveillance program for detection of dysplasia. The researchers found that the prevalence of colonic dysplasia was significantly decreased when ursodiol was used. This effect persisted after adjustment for sex, age at onset of colitis, duration of colitis and sclerosing cholangitis, severity of hepatic disease, and sulfasalazine use. Multivariate analysis revealed that age at onset, but not duration, of colitis independently influenced the risk of dysplasia.

39. Tale of Two Bugs: One Causes Cancer, One Kills it (Cancer Info—29/10/2000)

Not only is Campylobacter jejuni the most common cause of foodborne illness in the United States, but new research indicates it may contribute to intestinal cancer in those who consume it. Meanwhile, another study shows that

Salmonella, also a common cause of foodborne illness, may be used along with radiation to actually fight some forms of cancer.

It has been found that a protein toxin in Campylobacter may help the bacteria to colonize the intestine and then damage the DNA, making Campylobacter infection a possible predisposing factor for intestinal cancer. These findings are significant because little is known about how these bacteria cause disease and the research may lead to the development of novel therapeutic strategies and stimulate additional research.

40. Olive Oil may Protect against Colon Cancer (Times of India—20/09/2000)

Olive oil has been added to the list of foods that may help to prevent colon cancer. Comparison of cancer rates, diets and olive oil consumption in 28 countries including Europe, Britain, US, Brazil, Columbia, Canada and China have shown that olive oil is as good as fresh fruit and vegetables in keeping colon cancer at bay.

Researchers suspect olive oil protects against bowel cancer by influencing metabolism of the gut. They think it cuts the amount of deoxycyclic acid and regulated the enzyme diamine oxidase which may be linked to cell division in the bowel.

41. Intestinal Cancer (Times of India—22/08/2000)

Physical activity may protect men from intestinal ulcers. Although many people become infected with Helicobacter pylori, which causes ulcers, very few actually develop ulcers. Lifestyle factors such as smoking, alcohol consumption and psychological stress seem to play an additional role.

This is one of the few studies to explore the possible beneficial effects of physical activity on ulcers while considering age, smoking habits, alcohol use, body mass index and psychological tension to assess the efficacy of thalidomide and irinotecan in a larger group of patients with colorectal cancer.

42. Colorectal Cancer (Times of India—01/08/2000)

Colonoscopy detects colon cancer better than other

methods. Researchers investigated the benefits of using the most comprehensive type of screening for colorectal cancer in people without any symptoms. They used colonoscopy, where a tiny camera is threaded into the body through the rectum to view the entire colon or large intestine. Over 3000 healthy individuals between 50 and 75 were studied. 10% were found to have colon cancer or serious pre-cancerous growths. Sigmoidoscopy which views only the lower portion of the colon, would have missed a third of these growths.

Colonoscopy has proved to be superior to barium enema in cancer screening. In a 10 year follow-up study, 580 patients who already had some small growths called polyps removed from their colons, underwent both a barium enema and a colonoscopy. The barium enema could only detect a third of the polyps detected through colonoscopy. It also detected only half of the polyps larger than one centimeter, which are likely to become cancerous.

43. FDA Approves Camptosar (Irinotecan Hydrochloride) in Combo Therapy for Metastatic Colorectal Cancer (Cancer Info—26/04/2000)*

Pharmacia Corporation announced that the U.S. Food and Drug Administration (FDA) approved Camptosar(R) (irinotecan hydrochloride injection), as first-line therapy for the treatment of patients with metastatic colorectal cancer (advanced cancer that has spread beyond the colon or rectum) in combination with 5-fluorouracil/leucovorin (5-FU/LV).

44. Everything you Need to Know about Colon Cancer and How to Prevent It (Time Europe—20/03/00)*

Colon cancer is one of the deadliest and most preventable malignancies. This article covers what you need to know about the disease and the surprisingly painless test that could save your life. Many people would prefer to ignore the fact that cancers of the large intestine, which includes the colon and the rectum, are relatively common and can be deadly. According to the London-based Cancer Research Campaign, colorectal cancer kills 98,500 men and women each year in the European Union, and among men it is the second most common cause of death from cancer. Although it occurs more frequently after the age of 50, younger people are also affected. Over the next 12 months, an estimated 437,000 people worldwide will die of the disease. But the good news is, it doesn't have to be this way. Provided it's caught in its earliest, most treatable stages, colorectal cancer is curable more than 90% of the time. "This is a disease almost no one needs to die from," says Carolyn Aldigé, President of the Cancer Research Foundation of America.

If more people underwent routine screening to find small tumors, experts estimate, the death toll could drop by 50% to 75%. Early detection works, treatment is improving and what you eat and how you exercise can dramatically reduce your chances of developing the disease.

There are probably more myths and misconceptions about colon cancer than about any other killer disease. Young people think only old people get it. Women think only men get it. In fact, the disease strikes men and women, young and old. And the rest of us—mired in inhibitions that date back to our toilet training—don't even want to think about it. Potty talk is for two-year-olds, not grown-ups. The idea of a full-scale colon exam (You're going to stick that thing where?) scares most people away from the very screening test that could save their life.

Nearly all colon cancers start as polyps, tiny grapelike projections that sprout on the inside of the large intestine.

45. Doctors Develop Blood Test for Colorectal Cancer (Medivision—15-31 December)

A new blood test developed by doctors in Philadelphia could give people with colorectal cancer a clearer idea of whether their disease is likely to spread or return after surgery, a study suggests.

The test can detect the spread of cancer from the intestine to the lymph nodes by searching the blood for a protein called guanylyl cyclase C or GCC, one of seven proteins made only by intestinal cells and colorectal cancer cells.

46. Value of Prostate Cancer Screening Unclear: Panel (Reuters—03/12/2002)

Screening for prostate cancer provides only uncertain benefits, a US government panel found, saying there was not enough evidence to recommend for or against men undergoing routine tests. The report's findings, based on a review of studies of the effect of screening for the disease, the second-leading cancer killer of US men after lung cancer, add to a growing debate on the subject. "While the jury is still out on the value of routine screening to improve health outcomes, patients should talk with their clinicians to make individualized decisions," Alfred Berg, head of the panel and chair of the University of Washington's Department of Family Medicine, said in a statement. "Men will need to make this decision based on their personal preferences and values until we have better scientific evidence on whether screening is effective."

Men who are diagnosed with prostate cancer and do decide on treatment may undergo surgery or radiation therapy that can leave them impotent, incontinent or with bowel dysfunction. "Older men and men with other significant medical problems who have a life expectancy of fewer than 10 years are unlikely to benefit from screening," the report said.

47. Study: Garlic May Prevent Cancer (AP—06/11/2002)

Men in China have the lowest rate of prostate cancer in the world, and a diet rich in garlic, shallots and onions may be one of the reasons. Researchers at the National Cancer Institute report in a new study that a diet with lots of vegetables from the allium food group—which includes garlic, shallots and onions—reduces the risk of prostate cancer by about half. And the common Chinese diet includes hearty servings of these vegetables. Men who are interested in preventing prostate cancer should make sure that their diet includes plenty of garlic, scallions, chives and other vegetables in the allium family. Previous research has also linked the intake of allium vegetables to a lower risk of stomach, colon and esophagus cancer. These vegetables are rich in the anti-oxidants known as flavonols and other compounds that have been found to inhibit tumor growth in laboratory studies.

Scallions seemed to be the most protective. According to

the study, men who ate about a tenth of an ounce or more a day of scallions reduced their prostate cancer risk by about 70 percent. For garlic consumption of the same amount, the prostate cancer risk was reduced by about 53 percent. Hsing said that the typical Chinese diet is much more heavily seasoned with garlic, scallions and onions than is the traditional American diet. But even so, the amount of allium vegetables consumed is measured only in fractional ounces. For instance, the study suggests that an effective level of prostate cancer protection can be achieved with about one clove of garlic a day. "The reduced risk of prostate cancer associated with allium vegetables was independent of body size, intake of other foods and total calorie intake," the study authors reported. Hsing said the study reinforces earlier studies that have linked high vegetable consumption to a reduced risk of prostate cancer.

For instance, earlier studies have found that eating tomatoes and tomato products can lower risk of prostate cancer. Italy, where tomato sauce and garlic are favorites, has one of the lowest rates of prostate cancer in Europe, said Hsing. Janet Stanford, a cancer epidemiologist at the Fred Hutchinson Cancer Research Center in Seattle, said the study by Hsing and her co-authors continues to support the general finding that "eating vegetables is a good thing." Stanford said her group, in an earlier study, linked broccoli, cauliflower and related vegetables to a reduced prostate cancer risk, while a high fat diet increased the risk. "This shows that your mother was right," said Stanford. "Eat more vegetables."

48. Prostate Cancer Patients Back Screening Program (Reuters—04/10/2002)

Men suffering from prostate cancer support screening programs to detect early signs of the disease, although the jury is still out on whether testing saves lives, doctors said. Medical experts are debating the evidence on the prostate specific antigen or PSA test, which measures levels of a molecule that is over-produced by cancerous prostate cells. PSA testing can detect the disease before symptoms occur. But research has shown that men may be getting unnecessary treatment because they would have died of something else, and there is conflicting evidence about whether testing reduces deaths from the disease. But most British men with the illness say they would recommend it for their friends and sons and believe a national screening program would encourage men to be tested.

49. Early Surgery Shown to Cut Prostate Cancer Deaths (Reuters Health—11/09/02)

In findings expected to help answer the long-debated question of how to treat early prostate cancer, new research shows that prostate removal does cut men's risk of dying from the disease. What's more, researchers say, although such surgery often carries significant side effects including impotence and incontinence, patients' overall quality of life after surgery may be no different from that of men who opt for "watchful waiting." The question of whether to aggressively treat early prostate cancer is controversial, due to both the nature of the disease and the risks of treatment.

It is estimated that by the time they reach age 75, at least half of men have some cancerous changes in their prostates, while up to one-third of men may have microscopic signs of the disease at age 50. But far fewer will actually die of prostate cancer. Watchful waiting means that when cancer is detected, no immediate treatment is given, and the patient is instead monitored for signs that his prostate cancer is progressing. The approach is based on the premise that early prostate cancer may grow so slowly that it will never become a serious health threat; studies have shown that men with early cancer confined to the prostate gland can live years without signs of disease. But in the US, the past two decades have seen a sharp increase in surgery to remove the prostate gland—referred to as radical prostatectomy—despite the fact that it has been unclear whether it extends the lives of men with cancer confined to the prostate.

50. High-Fat Diet May Foster Prostate Cancer Spread (Reuters Health—02/09/2002)

New research has linked a high-fat, high-calcium diet to an increased risk of advanced prostate cancer. And higher total calorie intake, the researchers found, appeared to boost the risk of both localized and more advanced prostate cancer. This suggests that modifying diet after prostate cancer treatment could help reduce the risk that cancer will return, according to Dr. Alan Kristal from the Fred Hutchinson Cancer Research Center in Seattle, Washington, and colleagues. "Our findings clearly show decreased risk for late-stage disease in men with diets that are low in fat and moderate in calcium, perhaps because these diets slow progression of prostate cancer into more aggressive disease," Kristal said in a statement. "For men diagnosed with early-stage prostate cancer, this finding could be important because it suggests that moderating fat and calcium consumption may reduce the risk of cancer recurrence following treatment," he added.

51. Surgery, Radiotherapy Equivalent for Localized Prostate Cancer (Reuters Health—30/08/2002)

For patients with clinically localized prostate cancer, radical prostatectomy and external-beam radiotherapy are equally effective, results of a single-center study suggest. Dr. Patrick A. Kupelian, now of M.D. Anderson Cancer Center Orlando, and colleagues at the Cleveland Clinic determined biochemical relapse-free survival rates for 1054 men who underwent radical prostatectomy and 628 who underwent external-beam radiotherapy for localized prostate cancer. Eight-year biochemical relapse-free survival rates for surgery and radiotherapy were similar, 72% and 70%, respectively, the team reports in the *Journal of Clinical Oncology*.

52. Findings Support PSA Tests for High-Risk Men (Reuters Health—09/08/2002)

French scientists say their research findings support targeted prostate cancer screenings for men with a family history of the disease. Currently, the American Cancer Society recommends annual prostate specific antigen (PSA) testing and a rectal exam beginning at age 50—and at age 45 for African Americans and men with a family history of the disease, who face a higher risk. Several other scientific and medical groups do not recommend routine prostate cancer screening.

PSA is a protein produced by the prostate gland. PSA levels above 4 nanograms per milliliter (ng/mL) of blood can signal prostate cancer, but not always—sometimes a rise in PSA is due to another cause, and sometimes cancer can occur without a rise in PSA.

53. Adding Androgen Suppression to Radiotherapy Improves Prostate Cancer Survival (Reuters Health—12/07/2002)

In patients with locally advanced prostate cancer, radiotherapy plus immediate androgen suppression provides significantly better survival outcomes than radiotherapy alone, according to a report published in *The Lancet*. Dr. Michel Bolla, from the University Hospital in Grenoble, France, and colleagues assessed the outcomes of 415 patients.

54. Living with Prostate Cancer (Health Scout News—07/07/2002)

No wonder the mention of prostate cancer makes many men shudder. It's the second leading cause of cancer deaths in American men, exceeded only by lung cancer. However, if detected early, it's a very treatable cancer, even though the exact cause isn't known and the side effects of some therapies can diminish a man's quality of life. About 189,000 new cases of prostate cancer will be diagnosed in American men this year, the American Cancer Society says. Upon diagnosis, most men have a range of treatment options, from surgery to radiation to hormone therapy. The best choice depends on their age, health and concerns about side effects. In general, surgery or radiation treatment continue to be the best options, says Dr. Arnold Kwart, chairman of the urology department at the Washington Hospital Center in Washington, D.C. "Drug or hormone treatments are, by and large, palliatives," Kwart says. "If they're curative, they're curative may be in about 10 percent of patients."

"The secret is picking it up early," he says.

55. It's Prostate Cancer—Or is it? (Health Scout News—02/07/2002)

A large number of men who are given the scary news that they have prostate cancer are being rattled—and perhaps treated—unnecessarily, a new study suggests. The diagnosis for those men is based on detection of high levels of prostate-specific antigen (PSA), a molecule associated with the malignancy. The computer study concludes that many of them—29 percent of whites, 44 percent of blacks—would be better-off not knowing that diagnosis because they would die of other causes before the cancer did any damage. PSA testing was approved by the U.S. Food and Drug Administration in 1986 as a way to monitor treatment of prostate cancer.

The model was based on a hypothetical group of men aged 60 to 84. The estimated percentages of over-diagnoses (higher for blacks than whites because they are more susceptible to the cancer, for unknown reasons) were based on two factors: Either the cancer would grow so slowly that it would not affect a young man, or an older man would die of other causes before the cancer caused a problem. Unfortunately, the model provides no guidance for a man who is told his PSA level is high enough to require treatment.

56. Clues on Vitamin E's Anti-Prostate Cancer Effects (Reuters Health—29/05/2002)

Vitamin E appears to protect against prostate cancer, and new research shows it may do so by interfering with two proteins that are associated with the disease. Researchers based at the University of Rochester in New York found that adding Vitamin E to prostate cancer cells inhibits the production of a receptor for testosterone, called the androgen receptor (AR), which is needed in order for the cancer to grow and develop. "The fewer ARs there are in a (prostate cancer) cell, the less capable the remaining ARs, no matter how they are activated, are to turn on the genes that stimulate (prostate cancer) growth and progression," study author Dr. Edward M. Messing told Reuters Health. "Thus, this can be combined with other AR inhibiting strategies to eliminate AR activity in (prostate cancer) cells," he added.

57. Putting Cancer in Deep Freeze (Health Scout News—17/05/2002)

Doctors have been freezing malignant tumors for years with cryosurgery, but hardy cancer cells sometimes resist the arctic blasts and stay inside the body to cause more trouble later. Now researchers say a combination of cryosurgery and chemotherapy may wipe out all the malignant cells. "Cryosurgery is a very effective method for treatment of cancer, and it will become more effective," predicts study author Boris Rubinsky, a professor of bioengineering and mechanical engineering at the University of California, Berkeley. "I anticipate that some doctors will use this procedure as soon as this study goes into print." Doctors began to freeze tumors in the 1960s, but they were hampered by not being able to see inside the body. The procedure has become more common as scientists have developed probes that direct liquid nitrogen or argon gas to freeze tumors inside the body, and ultrasound machines now show doctors where they're going.

Doctors use cryosurgery to treat prostate cancer and liver cancer. Experiments are being done on pancreatic cancer and bone cancer.

58. Prostate on Course to Become Top UK Male Cancer (Reuters—28/05/2002)

Prostate cancer is on course to become the most common men's cancer in Britain in the next 3 years, health experts said. Cases of the disease have doubled in the past 20 years and scientists predict the numbers will continue to rise as the population ages and more men are tested for the illness. "The incidence of prostate cancer in this country has increased more rapidly than we had expected," Professor Colin Cooper told a news conference. The head of Britain's first dedicated male cancer research unit at The Institute of Cancer Research described the disease as an enigma. Although more men are being diagnosed with the disease, fewer are dying from it. Up to two-thirds of men with the illness may also not need treatment, which can cause side effects such as impotence and incontinence, but scientists do not know enough about the disease to determine whether or not a patient has an aggressive cancer. "What this means in reality is that many men could receive treatment who may not need it. On the other hand, if prostate cancer is not detected early by PSA testing, some men will have developed advanced, incurable disease," according to Dr. David Dearnaley, a male cancer expert at the institute.

59. Love can Conquer Impotence: One Couple's Story (Health Scout—26/03/2002)

For Virginia and Keith Laken, treating Keith's prostate cancer was just the beginning. "We had to redefine ourselves as to how our sexual relationship was going to be, and Keith had to redefine himself regarding his manliness," says Virginia, a communications consultant. "You need to understand that that's normal, that you're going to most likely need help with that." The Minnesota couple had been married more than 25 years and were enjoying their new empty nest when Keith was diagnosed with prostate cancer at the age of 49.

The Lakens advise couples confronting impotence to:

- communicate and candidly share information with each other,
- recognize the need to treat the mind as well as the body; seek help from support groups and mental health experts, and
- accept that emotional states can swing from high to low unexpectedly, especially during the first year of recovery.

60. Painkillers may Prevent Prostate Cancer (Times of India Online—12/03/2002)

Regular use of Aspirin, Ibuprofen and other common painkillers appear to protect against prostate cancer among older men, Mayo Clinic researchers said. Men over age 60 who took a daily dose of one of the drugs known collectively as non-steroidal anti-inflammatory drugs (NSAIDs) were half as likely to develop the disease, which is the second-leading cancer killer among US men with more than 30,000 deaths expected this year.

61. Tomato Products Reduce Risk of Prostate Cancer (Associated Press—06/03/2002)

A diet rich in tomato sauce, ketch-up and other tomato-based products containing a powerful anti-oxidant can lower the risk of prostate cancer, a new study says. Researchers analysed the food choices and prostate cancer histories of more than 47,000 men and found that those who ate at least two meals a week containing tomato products lowered their risk of prostate cancer by 24 to 36 per cent. Dr Edward Giovannucci of Brigham and Women's Hospital and the Harvard School of Public Health, the first author of the study, said it supports earlier research involving foods, particularly tomato products, that were high in lycopene, a powerful anti-oxidant. A report on the study appears in the Journal of the *National Cancer Institute.*

62. Biotech Firm Claims has found Potential Cancer Drug (Times of India Online—10/10/2001)

Myriad Genetics Inc., a biotechnology company that studies genes and proteins to discover new drugs, said it has found a way to kill a wide range of cancer cells without damaging healthy cells. Salt Lake City-based Myriad said its MPI-176716 compound causes cell death in several cancers, including prostate cancer and T-cell lymphoma. The target for MPI-176716 is a protein that has not been explored previously, the company said. If the human body is working as it should, normal cells are destroyed after they serve their function. If this process is damaged, cells may continue to divide and grow, resulting in cancer. Myriad said it has found a way to induce cells to destroy themselves if they are not doing it naturally. The company said the process may help it develop drugs that don't harm healthy cells, causing the kind of toxic side effects seen in treatments such as chemotherapy or radiation.

63. Insider's View into Cancer may Improve Treatments (Times of India Online—19/06/2001)

British researchers said on Sunday they have developed a new technique that could improve the accuracy and effectiveness of radiotherapy treatments for cancers and reduce harmful side effects. It combines two widely used scanning techniques, computed tomography (CT) and magnetic resonance imaging (MRI), to create computer-generated images of cancerous tumors. The technique will initially be used for radiotherapy for prostate cancer patients, but it could be helpful in treating other tumors, particularly in the pelvis, head and neck.

64. Men who Eat Soy and Tomatoes Reduce their Risk of Prostate Cancer, Study Shows (Cancer Info—09/06/2001)

Men at risk of prostate cancer might want to include more tofu and soy milk in their diets. Although the study was conducted with mice, and results must be replicated with humans, researchers found that a chemical found in soy slowed prostate cancer growth in mice and caused prostate cancer cells to die.

The soy chemical found to reduce prostate cancer in mice is called genistein, one of two compounds in soy that belong to a family of chemicals known as isoflavones. Isoflavones are phytoestrogens, plant-based chemicals that mimic the effects of estrogen in the body.

65. Oily Fishes Reduce Chances of Prostate Cancer (Times of India Online—02/06/2001)

Eating even moderate amounts of oily fish such as mackerel, salmon and sardines might reduce the risk of prostate cancer in half, new research suggests. Omega-3 fatty acids, plentiful in dark, oily fish, are known to fight heart diseases. They also have shown promise in protecting against cancers of colon, rectum and ovary. Previous studies have shown fatty fish oils can impede the growth of prostate cancer cells in laboratory dishes and in animals. In another study, prostate cancer was found less frequently in men who had high levels of fatty acids in their blood. Now, a new study, published this week in *The Lancet* medical journal, found that Swedish men who ate greasy fish only occasionally or not at all were twice as likely to develop prostate cancer as those who made it a moderate or large part of their diet.

67. High Boron Intake may cut Prostate Cancer Risk (Times of India Online—08/04/2001)

A new study suggests that men who consume high levels of boron—an element found in fruits and nuts—reduce their risk of prostate cancer. The study compared the diets of 76 men diagnosed with prostate cancer to the diets of 7,751 healthy males. All of the men completed 1-day dietary recall surveys.

Quercetin, a natural substance found in apples, onions, tea and red wine, may be a potentially novel approach for preventing and treating prostate cancer, according to a laboratory research study. Laboratory results showed quercetin blocks the androgen (hormone) activity in androgen-responsive human prostate cancer cell lines. By blocking the androgen activity, the growth of prostate cancer cells can be prevented or stopped. The study suggests quercetin may be a potential non-hormonal approach to accomplishing that goal.

67. Popular Herbal Compound Causes Prostate Cancer Cells to Die, Study Finds (Cancer Info—09/10/2000)

Researchers from Columbia University in New York and Henry Mondor Hospital in France measured the effects of PC-SPES, a compound consisting of eight herbs, on three different human prostate cancer cell lines, on human tumors implanted in mice and in a group of 69 men with prostate cancer. Since it first became commercially available in 1996, scientists have been studying PC-SPES, which as an herbal remedy is not regulated by the Food and Drug Administration. While there is a broad consensus that the mixture appears to mimic the actions of estrogens—and therefore counters the impact of tumor-fueling male hormones—investigators haven't been able to determine exactly how PC-SPES works against prostate cancer.

68. Chemoprevention for Prostate Cancer Looks to Drugs, Anti-oxidants (Cancer Info—28/03/00)

As the average age of Americans rises, preventing prostate cancer is becoming a vital area of research, and the focus is turning from general recommendations about diet, such as eating less fat and more fruits and vegetables, to exploring specific agents, including vitamins and drugs. About 30 percent of men between ages 30 and 39 have at least some cancer cells in their prostate, and that number rises to 50 percent for men in their fifties, said William G. Nelson, M.D., a medical oncologist at Johns Hopkins University Hospital in Baltimore. "It's a staggering thought, even as the population gets older on average," he added. To prevent these indolent cancers from turning aggressive, scientists are exploring the effects of a variety of substances, ranging from chemotherapeutic drugs used for other cancers to substances found in foods. At the Advances in Human Breast and Prostate Cancer Conference here recently, researchers discussed this burgeoning area of research called chemoprevention. One of the more promising possible chemopreventive agents comes from a class of drugs called selective estrogen receptor modulators (SERMs). These are thought to act by plugging into certain proteins on the surface of cells, thereby preventing estrogen from binding to those same sites and promoting cell growth. Blake Lee Neubauer, Ph.D., is one researcher looking at a specific SERM with the minimalist name LY353381-HCI to explore its potential for preventing the growth and spread of prostate cancer. It's already being tested in Phase II randomized trials for women with breast cancer, and considering the hormone-based growth of prostate cancer, it's being investigated for use in men with that disease as well.

Also of potential relevance to the prevention of prostate cancer is a collection of agents ranging from a substance found in tomatoes, to vitamins. Among the major cancers, prostate cancer is the least understood from an epidemiological point of view, observed Ronald Ross, M.D., an epidemiologist from the University of Southern California in Los Angeles, "which makes it difficult to target prevention pathways."

Some substances that merit future research in Ross's view are anti-oxidants, androgen suppressors and Vitamin D. "Each of the pathways [these substances affect] has several biological goals in common," he said, which are decreasing cellular proliferation, increasing cellular differentiation (return to a normal mature form), increasing apoptosis (programmed cell death) and decreasing mutations. Based on a 1993 study out of the California-based Kaiser-Permanente group, there's evidence supporting Vitamin D as a chemopreventive agent, Ross said. But scientists are still working out how to prevent hypercalcemia, a common side effect of taking too much of the vitamin. The anti-oxidants include selenium, lycopenes and vitamin E. Anti-oxidants neutralize free radicals, which can cause potentially cancer-stimulating DNA mutations.

LUNG CANCERS

69. Gene May Help Predict Lung Cancer Patient Survival (Reuters Health—20/11/2002)

Patients with lung cancer are more likely to survive longer if they have high levels of a protein produced by a so-called "repair gene," scientists told a cancer drug meeting. In a study of patients who had undergone surgery for the most common type of lung cancer, known as non-small-cell lung cancer, the investigators found that those with high levels of the protein had the longest survival time. "Currently, every patient with lung cancer gets the same treatment, chemotherapy, and surgery when possible," said Dr. Gerold Bepler, a professor of medicine and oncology at the University of South Florida in Tampa. "However, we can't predict who will respond to chemotherapy and what factors are associated with survival of lung cancer. If this gene turns out to be a reliable predictor, we could tell which patients could do without chemotherapy, and which ones should get it."

70. Cancer Trial to Test Whether CT Scans Save Lives (Health Scout News—18/09/2002)

The newest generation of CT scans can spot lung tumors when they are smaller and, presumably, more treatable. But do they save lives? Common sense would dictate a "yes" answer, but research hasn't proven that yet and some small studies have suggested they don't. The federal government intends to find out once and for all, announcing today that it is launching the biggest and most ambitious study yet to learn whether the high-tech scanners will actually cut the death rate from lung cancer.

Much is at stake because of the disease's toll. Were lung cancer a specific cause of death (officially, it's listed along with all other cancers), it would be the nation's third-leading killer. The disease will claim about 160,000 American lives this year, more than cancers of the breast, prostate, colon, and ovary combined. Another 160,000 or so Americans will be diagnosed with the disease this year. The NCI says that 87 percent of these patients smoke or used to smoke, and Gohagan says there are 90 million current or former smokers in this country.

Lung cancer is so deadly because it's not usually symptom-specific until it has already done significant damage. A patient often goes to the doctor with a cough, for instance, and an X-ray or CAT scan confirms the presence of a tumor. By that time, the cancer is well established in the lung and perhaps other parts of the body.

71. Breath Test has Potential for Lung Cancer Detection (Reuters Health—16/09/2002)

Tests of breath condensate can identify mutations of a cancer-suppressing gene in patients with lung cancer, a study presented at the Annual Congress of the European Respiratory Society demonstrates. This suggests that the method could one day be used to help identify lung cancer in its early stages, said Dr. Christian Gessner of the University of Leipzig, who presented the research at the meeting.

72. New Radiotherapy Regimen Ups Lung Cancer Survival (Reuters Health—04/09/2002)

Treating lung cancer patients with a higher dose of radiotherapy but giving them weekends off to recover can improve tumor control and increase survival rates, according to the results of a new study. Cancer Research UK scientists said computer models predicted that the new regimen could eradicate 33% of non-small-cell lung tumors compared with 19% under the current "gold standard" treatment system. Continuous hyperfractionated accelerated radiotherapy (CHART)—the present gold standard—gives patients three doses of radiation a day for 12 consecutive days. The new regimen, dubbed CHARTWEL, builds on CHART by giving a higher dose of radiation but one that is still tolerable and that incorporates a break at weekends

73. UA to Test Selenium use to Keep Disease at Bay (Arizona Daily Star—03/08/2002)

What if taking a single, inexpensive pill once a day could stop the most deadly of all cancers—lung cancer—in its tracks? That's the end of the research rainbow now getting under way at the University of Arizona. It may not be known for years if taking a daily dose of the trace mineral selenium can help prevent lung cancer in those at high risk for it—former smokers—but UA researchers have launched the first study to find out. During the next year, some 200 people with a long history of smoking—but who have now quit—will be given selenium or an inactive placebo pill. They will then be tested to see if lung damage that leads to cancer has been stopped or even reversed in those taking the selenium.

And that is where selenium is now when it comes to battling both colon and prostate cancers. After showing significant effectiveness in early studies, it is now being given to thousands of patients nationwide at high risk for those cancers, with funding from the National Cancer Institute.

74. Screen May Detect High-Risk Lung Cancer (Reuters Health—15/07/2002)

Michigan scientists have developed a method of identifying which patients with early-stage lung cancer might benefit most from aggressive treatment. Though the screening, which looks for genetic markers of aggressive cancer in tumor cells, is not yet ready for widespread use, the analysis eventually may help patients with high-risk cancers live longer, according to researcher Dr. David G. Beer.

"Targeting this gene product as a form of therapy for cancer is an active area of research in the scientific community."

75. Venting Stoves Cut Lung Cancer Rate in China (Reuters Health—05/06/2002)

Changing from unvented to vented coal-burning stoves appears to have reduced new cases of lung cancer in one region of China known for high rates of the disease, according to a recent report. In the past, residents of rural Xuanwei County in Yunnan Province typically used unvented indoor firepits or stoves for cooking and heating. Use of these stoves was associated with very high levels of indoor air pollution. During the 1970s, however, most residents changed to stoves with chimneys. Given that high levels of indoor air pollution are a risk factor for lung cancer, Dr. Robert S. Chapman from the US Environmental Protection Agency, Research Triangle Park, North Carolina, and colleagues decided to compare lung cancer rates in Xuanwei before and after the widespread use of vented stoves.

76. Aspirin May Cut Risk of Lung Cancer Risk—Study (Reuters—25/06/2002)

Aspirin, the century-old drug that relieves headaches and helps to prevent heart attacks and strokes, may also cut the risk of developing lung cancer, scientists said. Smoking is the cause of most cases of lung cancer but researchers at New York University School of Medicine have discovered that taking aspirin regularly may have a protective effect against the disease, which is a top cancer killer. "Not smoking is by far the best way to avoid lung cancer, but our study suggests that regular aspirin use could also confer some degree of protection against the disease.

77. New Pill May Improve Lung Cancer (Associated Press—19/05/2002)

A once-a-day pill that slows cancer by jamming its internal growth signals shows encouraging benefits in terminally ill lung cancer patients, quickly easing symptoms for many. Research showed that the drug, called Iressa, can shrink tumors in some patients who have failed all other therapy. But perhaps even more important for these patients, it relieves cancer symptoms in one-third or more of cases. The drug, not yet approved for routine use, is one of the new class of so-called targeted therapies that works by specifically interfering with cancer rather than all fast-growing tissue, as standard chemotherapy does. As a result, it carries far fewer side effects, and patients often can safely take it for months or even years. Many experts doubt that Iressa and drugs like it will actually cure cancer alone, but they say it may help hold the disease in check—especially if given in early stages. "This is a whole new way of treating lung cancer," said Dr. Mark Kris of Memorial Sloan-Kettering Cancer Center in New York City. "People didn't think this would work. It's nothing short of amazing."

Most who responded began to feel better within two weeks. The drug relieved their shortness of breath, coughs, poor appetites and other cancer symptoms. Symptom relief ranged from moderate to dramatic. "The patients felt the improvement was significant to them. It translated to a better quality of life," she said.

78. Study Ties Lung Cancer, Air Pollution (Yahoo News—05/03/2002)

Long-term exposure to the air pollution in some of America's biggest metropolitan areas significantly raises the risk of dying from lung cancer and is about as dangerous as living with a smoker, a study of a half-million people found. The study echoes previous research and provides the strongest evidence yet of the health dangers of the pollution levels found in many big cities and even some smaller ones, according to the researchers from Brigham Young University and New York University. The risk is from what scientists call combustion-related fine particulate

Lung cancer kills more than a million people worldwide each year and is now the leading cause of death from cancer among both men and women. Smoking causes the vast majority of cases.

79. Chemicals in Broccoli can cut Lung Cancer Risk (Cancer Info—23/09/2000)

New evidence from a large study in China suggests that chemicals contained in broccoli, cabbage, or bok choy can help protect people from developing lung cancer. The study of more than 18,000 men found that people with detectable amounts of chemicals known as isothiocyanates in their bodies had a 36% lower chance of developing lung cancer over 10 years than those without the chemicals. The chemicals are found in broccoli and other so-called "cruciferous" vegetables. Researchers from the National Institute of Environmental Health Sciences (NIEHS) in North Carolina along with colleagues in China performed the study in four small communities in Shanghai. That site is notable because of its population's high smoking rate and high level of cruciferous vegetable consumption, according to Dr. Stephanie J. London, an epidemiologist and the study's lead investigator.

While the results suggest that eating broccoli and related vegetables can lower cancer risk even for smokers, no one should assume that isothiocyanates would be enough to protect smokers from cancer. Though the chemicals did lower cancer risk by 36% in this study, smoking alone increases lung cancer risk by as much as 10 times.

80. Doctors Test New Vaccine for Lung Cancer (Cancer Info—20/07/2000)

Every 45 seconds, someone dies of lung cancer. In an effort to gain ground against this relentless killer, called the "epidemic of the 20th Century," a new vaccine is being tested which will is expected to stimulate the immune systems of lung cancer victims.

The stakes are high: While lung cancer survival rates have improved slightly, the increase in new cases wipes out the gains in numbers made fighting other types of cancer. Every third cancer death is from lung cancer, yet it is estimated that treatment advances lag 20 to 25 years behind that for breast cancer.

80. A Simple Way to Catch a Killer (TOI—03/02/00)

Pilot trials for a simple screening test that detects early stage lung cancer in smokers and ex-smokers show that it can lead to a remarkable five-fold increase in the number of people surviving one of the biggest cancer killers. One of the major obstacles in dealing with lung cancer successfully is that by the time patients get typical symptoms such as coughing, wheezing, etc., the tumor is often too big for surgery. As a result, overall survival rates are so dismal that only one in 10 of the new cases diagnosed this year will be alive five years from now. Most will die in the first year. But if diagnosed in the first stage, the survival rates soar to 70%. This potentially huge increase, coupled with an ability to easily target an identifiable at-risk group, smokers, makes it an ideal disease for screening. But very little has been done so far.

81. High Fat Diet and Lung Cancer (Health Notes—2002)

Some studies suggest an association between high blood or dietary levels of a particular dietary ingredient with a reduced risk of developing lung cancer. Common symptoms of cancer lung are: cough, the most common symptom of lung cancer, is likely to occur when a growing cancer blocks an airway. In some cases your saliva is streaked with rusty or even bright red blood. Another symptom is a chest pain. It occurs as a persistent ache that might or might not be related to coughing. You may develop a wheeze, or hoarseness, or find yourself short of breath. Repeat bouts of pneumonia or bronchitis, too may be an indication of lung cancer. And like all cancers, lung cancer can cause fatigue, loss of appetite, and weight loss. There are a number of tests he may use to confirm a suspected diagnosis of lung cancer and to determine the type of the disease.

Treatment of lung cancer may take several forms—surgery, radiation therapy, and chemotherapy often in combination, depending on your needs. Surgery is the most common treatment for cancers that are small, slow growing, and have neither invaded nearby tissue nor metastasized (spread). Your surgeon must determine how much of your lung to remove, and if it is necessary to include nearby lymph nodes (bean-shaped structures in the lymphatic system). Treatment by radiation therapy may be used in combination with surgery. It is given either before or after your operation. Radiation therapy may be administered in a number of ways. Chemotherapy (treatment with anti-cancer drugs) is available to your physician in treating lung cancer. Anti-cancer drugs kill cancer cells because the drugs can act on normal cells as well as cancerous ones, your physician must maintain a delicate balance of enough drugs to kill cancer cells without destroying too many healthy cells.

The following dietary changes have been studied in connection with lung cancer.

Rating	*Nutritional Supplements*	*Herbs*
★★★	Beta-carotene (reduces risk) Warning: Beta-Carotene increases the risk of lung cancer in smokers.	
★★☆	Selenium (reduces risk) Vitamin E (reduces risk)	Coriolus versicolor

★✯	Coenzyme Q10	Asian ginseng
	Folic acid (reduces risk)	Black tea (reduces risk)
	Melatonin	Dr. Sun's soup
	Multivitamins	Green tea (reduces risk)
	Vitamin A	Hoxsey Formula
	Vitamin B12 (reduces risk)	

Fruits and Vegetables

Most studies suggest that as consumption of fruits and vegetables increases, risk of lung cancer decreases. Flavonoids are found in virtually all fruits and vegetables. Onions and apples contain large amounts of a flavonoid called quercetin. Consumption of flavonoids in general, or quercetin-containing foods in particular, has been associated with a reduced risk of lung cancer. Tomatoes contain lycopene—an anti-oxidant similar in structure to beta-carotene. Lycopene has been reported to inhibit the proliferation of cancer cells in test tube research. Consumption of fried and well-done red meat was associated with an elevated risk of lung cancer in one report. Consumption of red meat in general, as well as fried meat, correlated with a high risk of lung cancer in another study. People who cook with fat taken from meat (such as bacon fat and lard) have also been reported to be at high risk of lung cancer according to preliminary research. Dietary cholesterol comes primarily from the consumption of eggs. Most but not all, 20 studies have reported that as dietary cholesterol increases, so does the risk of lung cancer. No clear explanation has yet emerged to account for this association. Fish-eaters have been reported to have low risks of many cancers including lung cancer. Preliminary studies have reported associations between an increasing intake of sugar or sugar-containing foods and an increased risk of several cancers including lung cancer. Whether this association exists because sugar directly promotes cancer or because sugar consumption is only a marker for some other dietary or lifestyle factor remains unknown.

Cigarette smoking is universally acknowledged to be the leading cause of lung cancer, both in the United States and worldwide. Many studies now show that exposure to passive smoke—the cigarette smoke from others' cigarettes—

significantly increases the risk of lung cancer. Inhalant exposure to diesel exhaust, pitch and tar, dioxin, arsenic, chromium, cadmium, and nickel compounds may also increase the risk of lung cancer. Exposure to asbestos is associated with an increased risk of lung cancer. Radon exposure has been reported to contribute to the risk of lung cancer in the general population.

Folic Acid and Vitamin B_{12}

Folic Acid and vitamin B_{12} work together in the body to help cells replicate normally. Synthetic beta-carotene supplementation has led to an increased risk of lung cancer in smokers, though not in groups consisting primarily of non-smokers. The researchers who conducted the lung cancer trials have been criticized for not having used the natural form of beta-carotene.

Selenium

Selenium has been reported to have diverse anti-cancer actions. Blood levels of selenium have been reported to be low in patients with many cancers, including lung cancer. Similarly, high blood levels and dietary levels of vitamin E have been associated with a reduced risk of lung cancer. In one trial, patients with very early stage lung cancer ("stage I") were all treated with surgery and then given either 300,000 IU of Vitamin A per day or no Vitamin A. After one year, 63% of those taking Vitamin A were free of cancer compared with 52% of those not assigned to Vitamin A. In patients with advanced lung cancer who were given 10 mg of melatonin at night in cycles of three weeks on followed by one week-off, survival time was almost twice as long as survival in those not given melatonin—a statistically significant increase.

Coenzyme Q10 Supplementation

In an unpublished report, 4 of 11 lung cancer patients were said to be alive following ten years of supplementation with 100 mg of CoQ_{10} per day. Some lung cancer patients have been reported to lose excessive amounts of zinc in urine. In one trial, supplementing such patients with zinc led to an improvement in some aspects of immunity. In a preliminary trial, lung cancer patients who reported using vitamin supplements survived almost four times as long as those who did not.

Cloud mushroom extracts, have been studied in preliminary and double-blind trials and shown to be beneficial in extending the life of patients with several.

Asian Ginseng (Panax Ginseng)

Many studies of animals with cancer suggest Asian ginseng may improve immune function and increase lifespan.

Green Tea and Black Tea studies have shown an association between drinking green tea and a reduced risk of several types of cancers.

Hoxsey formula as given below may also help to a variable extent.

- Potassium iodide
- Licorice *(Glycyrrhiza glabra)*
- Red clover *(Trifolium pratense)*
- Alder Buckthorn *(Rhamnus frangula)*
- Burdock *(Actrium lappa)*
- Stillingia root *(Stillingia sylvatica)*
- Barberry root *(Berberis vulgaris)*
- Poke root *(Phytolacca decandra)*
- Cascara amarga *(Picramnia antidesma)* or Cascara sagrada *(Rhamnus purshina)*
- Prickly ash *(Zanthoxylum fraxineum)*

Limited evidence suggests that some of the components of the Hoxsey formula may have anti-cancer activity.

CANCER PREVENTION AND DIET

Cancer is the second leading cause of death in Americans. Cancer refers to a large number of diseases categorized by unregulated replication of cells.

The contents of this article are limited to information about diet and to a discussion of cancer prevention—not treatment. Prevention of cancer in a person who has never had cancer is called "primary" prevention. Primary prevention is the focus of this article.

This article includes a discussion of studies that have assessed whether certain dietary ingredients may be beneficial in connection with the reduction of risk of developing cancer.

However, this information is provided solely to aid consumers in discussing such issues with their health care providers. It is not advised nor is this information intended to advocate, promote, or encourage self-use of this information for cancer risk reduction.

Finally, some of the studies suggest an association between high blood or dietary levels of a particular dietary ingredient with a reduced risk of developing cancer. Even if such an association were established, this does not mean that dietary supplements containing large amounts of the dietary ingredient will necessarily have a cancer risk reduction effect.

Prevention of a recurrence in a cancer patient who is in remission is called "secondary" prevention. Whether the information in this article would be helpful to people interested in secondary prevention is, for the most part, unknown. However, of cancer patients who are in complete remission, the information presented here is unlikely to help people who were ever diagnosed with metastatic cancer (also known as stage IV, or advanced, cancer).

Dietary changes that may be helpful: The following dietary changes have been studied in connection with cancer.

Alcohol and Cancer

Alcohol consumption significantly increases the risk of cancers of the mouth (oral/oropharyngeal cancer), throat (esophageal cancer), and voice box (laryngeal cancer), particularly in conjunction with cigarette smoking. Most studies documenting these associations also report that former drinkers have significantly lower risks for these cancers compared with current drinkers. Strong correlations between alcohol consumption and the risk of having liver cancer have also been reported.

Little is known about the effect of alcohol intake on the risk of female cancers other than breast cancer. Of the few published studies, findings have been inconsistent.

Fiber

Whole grains (such as rye, brown rice, and whole wheat contain high amounts of insoluble fiber—the type of fiber some scientists believe may help protect against a variety of cancers. In an analysis of the data from many studies, people who eat relatively high amounts of whole grains were reported to have low risks of lymphomas and cancers of the pancreas, stomach, colon, rectum, breast, uterus, mouth, throat, liver, and thyroid. Most research focusing on the relationship between cancer and fiber has focused on breast and colon cancers.

Consuming a diet high in insoluble fiber is best achieved by switching from white rice to brown rice and from bakery goods made with white flour or mixed flours to 100% whole wheat bread, whole rye crackers, and whole grain pancake mixes. Refined white flour is generally listed on food packaging labels as "flour," "enriched flour," "unbleached flour," "durum wheat," "semolina," or "white flour." Breads containing only whole wheat are often labeled "100% whole wheat."

Vegetarianism

The following two possibilities are both strongly

supported by research findings:

- Some foods consumed by vegetarians may protect against cancer.
- Eating meat may increase the risk of cancer.

Compared with meat-eaters, most, but not all, studies have found that vegetarians are less likely to be diagnosed with cancer. Vegetarians have also been shown to have stronger immune function, possibly explaining why vegetarians may be partially protected against cancer. Female vegetarians have been reported to have lower estrogen levels compared with meat-eating women, possibly explaining a lower incidence of uterine and breast cancers. A reduced risk for various cancers is only partly, not totally, explained by differences in body weight, smoking habits, and other lifestyle issues.

Fruits and Vegetables

Consumption of fruits and vegetables is widely accepted as lowering the risk of most common cancers. Many doctors recommend that people wishing to reduce their risk of cancer eat several pieces of fruit and several portions of vegetables every day. Optimal intakes remain unknown.

Most doctors also recommend that people should not consider supplements as substitutes for the real thing. Some of the anti-cancer substances found in produce have probably not yet been discovered, while others are not yet available in supplement form. More important, some research, particularly regarding synthetic beta-carotene, does not support the idea that taking supplements has the same protective value against cancer as does consumption of fruits and vegetables.

Flavonoids

Flavonoids are found in virtually all herbs and plant foods. Consumption of flavonoid-rich onions and apples contain large amounts of one flavonoid called quercetin. Consumption of flavonoids in general, or quercetin-containing foods in particular, has been associated with protection against cancer in some, but not all, preliminary studies.

Tomatoes

Tomatoes contain lycopene—an anti-oxidant similar in structure to beta-carotene. Most lycopene in our diet comes from tomatoes, though traces of lycopene exist in other foods. Lycopene inhibits the proliferation of cancer cells in test tube research.

A review of published research found that higher intake of tomatoes or higher blood levels of lycopene correlated with protection from cancer in 57 of 72 studies. Findings in 35 of these studies were statistically significant. Evidence of a protective effect for tomato consumption was strongest for cancers of the prostate, lung, and stomach, but some evidence of a protective effect also appeared for cancers of the pancreas, colon, rectum, esophagus (throat), mouth, breast, and cervix.

Cruciferous Vegetables

Cabbage, Brussels sprouts, broccoli, and cauliflower belong to the Brassica family of vegetables, also known as "cruciferous" vegetables. In test tube and animal studies, these foods have been associated with anti-cancer activity, possibly due to several substances found in these foods, such as indole-3-carbinol, glucaric acid (calcium D-glucarate), and sulforaphane. In a preliminary human study, people who ate cruciferous vegetables were reported to have a lower-than-average risk for bladder cancer.

Meat (how it is cooked) and Childhood Cancers

In one report, high consumption of hot dogs was associated with an almost tenfold increase in the risk of childhood leukemia when compared with low consumption. In another report, maternal consumption of hot dogs and childhood consumption of hamburgers or hot dogs at least once per week were associated with a doubling of the risk of cancers in children. A review of nine studies found an association between consumption by pregnant women of cured meat and the risk of brain cancer in their offspring. These associations do not yet constitute proof that eating hot dogs or hamburgers causes cancer in children, and evidence linking cured meat consumption to childhood cancers remains somewhat inconsistent.

In the report studying the effects of eating hot dogs and hamburgers, the association between meat eating and leukemia was weakest among children who took vitamin supplements. Processed meats, such as hot dogs, contain nitrates and nitrites-precursors to carcinogens. Anti-oxidants found in multivitamins keep nitrates and nitrites from converting into those carcinogens. Therefore, the association between vitamin consumption in children and protection against childhood cancers remains plausible, though unproven.

Fish

Fish-eaters have been reported to have low risks of cancers of the mouth, throat, stomach, colon, rectum, pancreas, lung, breast, and prostate. The omega-3 fatty acids found in fish are thought by some researchers to be the components of fish responsible for protection against cancer.

Coffee

Years ago, researchers reported the greater the consumption of coffee in a country, the higher the risk of pancreatic cancer in that country. An analysis of data from studies published between 1981 and 1993 did find some association between high consumption of coffee and an increased risk of pancreatic cancer. Surprisingly, however, the same report found that people drinking only one or two cups of coffee per day had, on average, a *lower* risk of pancreatic cancer compared with people who never drink coffee.

Most, but not all, published reports have shown coffee drinkers are at increased risk of bladder cancer, though in one case the relationship was found only in men. In another study, the association was found only with caffeinated coffee. A review of 35 trials found a small (7%) increased risk of bladder cancer in coffee drinkers compared with people not drinking coffee—a difference not statistically significant.

Calories

Scientists have known for many years that severe restriction of calories dramatically reduces the risk of cancer in laboratory animals. Scientists speculate that caloric content of the human diet may also affect cancer rates, though much less is known about the effect, if any, of moderate caloric restrictions in humans. In one report, adults with cancer were more likely to have consumed more calories during childhood compared with healthy adults. In other reports, attempts to find associations between reduced intake of calories and cancer have produced mixed results.

Only *severe* restriction in caloric intake provides significant protection in animal studies. As most people are unlikely to severely restrict calories, the association between caloric restriction and protection from cancer may ultimately prove to only be of academic interest.

Dietary Fat

In studying data from country to country, incidence of ovarian cancer correlates with dietary fat intake. According to preliminary research, consumption of saturated fat, dietary cholesterol (as found in eggs), and animal fat in general correlates with the risk of ovarian cancer.

Preliminary studies suggest dietary fat may correlate with the risk of uterine cancer. Some of the excess risk appears to result from increased body weight that results from a high-fat diet.

Many years ago, researchers reported that animals on a high-fat diet formed skin cancers more rapidly than did other animals. Although some preliminary human research has found no relationship between dietary fat intake and the risk of skin cancer, patients with basal cell and squamous cell skin cancers who were put on a low-fat diet for two years were reported to show a significant decrease in the number of new skin cancers compared with patients who maintained a high-fat diet. Similarly, pre-cancerous lesions of the skin have been prevented in people put on a low-fat diet.

Polyunsaturated Fats

A chain of carbon atoms in which several are not attached to the maximum possible amount of hydrogen is called "polyunsaturated"—in other words, unsaturated with hydrogen in several places. When nutrition researchers talk about polyunsaturated fatty acids, they are often referring primarily to linoleic acid—a fatty acid found in nuts and seeds and most vegetable oils.

In animal research, the consumption of polyunsaturated fatty acids increases the risk of some cancers. However, in humans, most, though not all, reports do not find an association between polyunsaturates and cancer risks.

Sugar

A preliminary study has reported an association between an increasing intake of sugar or sugar-containing foods and an increased risk of gallbladder cancer. Whether this association exists because sugar directly promotes cancer or because sugar consumption is only a marker for some other dietary or lifestyle factor remains unknown.

Salt

In preliminary research, increasing intake of salt correlates with increased risk of stomach cancer. Associations between foods preserved with salt and the risk of cancers of the head and neck have also been reported.

INDEX